Single-case and Small-*n* Experimental Designs

A Practical Guide to Randomization Tests

Second Edition

Single-case and Small-*n* Experimental Designs

A Practical Guide to Randomization Tests

Second Edition

Pat Dugard
Dundee University, UK

Portia File
University of Abertay Dundee, UK

Jonathan Todman
NHS Scotland

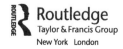
Routledge
Taylor & Francis Group
New York   London

Routledge
Taylor & Francis Group
711 Third Avenue
New York, NY 10017

Routledge
Taylor & Francis Group
2 Park Square, Mtlon Park
Abingdon, Oxon, OX14 4RN

© 2012 by Taylor & Francis Group, LLC
Routledge is an imprint of Taylor & Francis Group, an Informa business

International Standard Book Number: 978-0-415-88622-2 (Hardback) 978-0-415-88693-2 (Paperback)

Library of Congress Cataloging-in-Publication Data

Dugard, Pat.
    Single-case and small-n experimental designs : a practical guide to randomization
tests, second edition / Pat Dugard, Portia File, Jonathan Todman. -- 2nd ed.
       p. cm.
    Rev. ed. of: Single-case and small-n experimental designs / John B. Todman, Pat
Dugard. 2001.
    Summary: "Randomization tests are not a new idea, but they only became really
useful after the advent of fast computing. Making randomization tests accessible
to many more potential users by providing the means to use them within familiar
statistical software, this book serves as an introduction and provides macros to
perform in the familiar environments of SPSS and Excel. Though we expect that
the book will still appeal to researchers, we believe the changes in the new edition
will make the book an essential aid for graduate and senior undergraduate courses
in statistics, data analysis, and/or research methods, taught in departments of
psychology (especially clinical or counseling psychology), medicine, nursing, and
other health and social sciences"-- Provided by publisher.
    Includes bibliographical references and index.
    ISBN 978-0-415-88693-2 (pbk.) -- ISBN 978-0-415-88622-2 ()
    1. Statistical hypothesis testing. 2. Experimental design. I. File, Portia. II. Todman,
John B. III. Todman, John B. Single-case and small-n experimental designs. IV. Title.

QA277.T63 2011
519.5'6--dc23
                                          2011028087

Visit the Taylor & Francis Web site at
http://www.taylorandfrancis.com

and the Psychology Press Web site at
http://www.psypress.com

Dedication

To the memory of John Todman

Contents

Preface

This book is intended as a practical guide for students and researchers who are interested in the statistical analysis of data from single-case or very small-n experiments. We said this in the preface to the first edition, and it is true of this new edition as well. Randomization tests are not a new idea, but they became really useful only after the advent of fast computing. John Todman, lead author of the first edition of this book, wanted to make randomization tests accessible to many more potential users by providing the means to use them within familiar statistical software. As such, this book serves as an introduction to randomization tests and provides macros to perform some of them in the familiar environments of SPSS and Excel, which are already being used for data analysis by thousands of researchers. Minitab was dropped from this edition, because we believe fewer people are using it now, but the macros (plus a new one) for use with SPSS and Excel are still a central feature of the book. As well as the macros, we provide all the information you need to apply them to your own data.

Because most researchers are not familiar with randomization designs and tests, even if they are quite confident with data analysis and statistical inference, we have described the basic ideas of randomization tests using several extended examples. We also use examples to show how to choose a suitable design and, having made a choice, how to implement it and analyze the results. The emphasis throughout is on practical application and understanding when and how to use randomization tests. There is a book Web site (http://www.researchmethodsarena.com/9780415886932) from which you can take the macros and example data. There is a separate site for instructors only that contains the solutions to the exercises that are not included in the text.

If you are among that majority of researchers and students who are unfamiliar with randomization tests, studying this book will enable you to understand how randomization tests work, why they can be used in

many investigations that have too few participants for the familiar *t* tests or
ANOVAs, and why their use had to await readily available fast computing.
You will also learn how to choose, implement, and analyze randomization
designs. We provide the tools, instructions, and demonstration examples
for analysis in the familiar environment of SPSS or Excel. You will be able
to apply these techniques to your own investigations and data.

New to this edition

In the years since the original publication, many readers have contacted us
with queries, and we realized we had not gone far enough in explaining randomization tests to those who need to use them. So for this edition, we have
reordered and revised most of the text and introduced many new examples
from education and clinical research in psychology and medicine.

We have added exercises at the end of Chapters 2 to 7. Half of the solutions are provided at the back of the book for self-study, and the other half
are on the Instructor's Teaching Resource Web site (http://www.research-
methodsarena.com/9780415886932).

We have added an appendix to help with skills such as choosing a
random number, arranging objects in random order, listing and counting possible intervention points for phase designs, and checking for serial
correlation. Many readers may not have used these skills much but are
more familiar with taking random samples or random assignments to different conditions.

We have also added a glossary. The first time a technical term is used,
it appears in italics, and a brief definition can be found in the glossary (but
we also occasionally use italics for emphasis).

The first edition provided the macros on a CD, but for this edition they
can be taken from the book Web site along with example datasets. Readers
of the first edition will see that we have rationalized the names of the
macros, and the example data file names match them. We use screenshots
to show you how to use the macros and understand the results. We expect
that the more extended explanations, wider range of examples, exercises,
skills appendix, glossary, screenshots, and improved labeling of macros
and datasets will make this new edition a much better tool for students
and researchers who need randomization tests.

Though we expect that the book will still appeal to researchers, we
believe the changes in the new edition will make the book an essential aid
for graduate and senior undergraduate courses in statistics, data analysis,
and/or research methods, taught in departments of psychology (especially

clinical or counseling psychology), medicine, nursing, and other health and social sciences. We hope that clinicians, who are among those most likely to need single-case or small-n designs, will be empowered to use these techniques in their own work. For more ambitious readers who may want to adapt our macros or write their own, we have extended and improved the explanations for the macros, and (in Chapter 8) we have demonstrated how to tackle such an adaptation or extension. The macro listings with the new explanations are now in Appendices 2 and 3, one each for SPSS and Excel. We have rationalized the variable names in the macros, so the explanations are easier to follow. There is a new macro for a small-n repeated measures design with replicates, which we wrote in response to a reader query. Macro listings for you to use, without the explanations, are on the book Web site along with the example datasets so you don't have to type them out yourself.

We have done some updating for this edition, but the main difference you will notice is that we have made much more effort to help you to see how you might use the randomization tests we demonstrate and understand how they work. We assume some knowledge of ordinary statistical work and a little knowledge of nonparametric tests would be useful. A basic introduction to SPSS or Excel is also assumed so that you can use the macros for your own data, but we provide step-by-step instruction in using the macros in Chapter 4 and the Appendices.

Contents

Chapter 1 puts randomization tests into the context of investigations with human participants to show how they can fit into the research process. Of course, they can be used in other investigations, but it is when we have human participants that we are most likely to have a single case or just a few.

Chapter 2 demonstrates the main ideas used in the rest of the book with some examples of randomization tests. For many readers, these ideas will be new. Instead of basing inferences on random sampling, we use random assignment in the design and random reassignments for comparison with the experimental results.

In Chapter 3, we consider the ways in which our choice of design may be constrained, how we address internal and external validity in randomization designs, and how different methods of randomization may be used. We show how to choose a suitable design and list the key features of the designs covered.

Chapter 4 shows how to implement the chosen design. This includes how to do the randomization, and where necessary draws attention to potentially inappropriate randomization methods.

Chapter 5 demonstrates the analysis using the macros. There are instructions on using them for those who may not have used macros before, and screenshots to show the results using example data. We also show how the results could be reported.

Chapter 6 shows how randomization tests fit into the body of statistical inference, and also why using a randomization design may be worth the effort even if you intend to use only a graphical analysis.

Chapter 7 discusses power. This can be problematical for phase designs, and they receive special consideration.

Chapter 8 is for those who want to take these ideas further and perhaps even write their own macros. We use the process of writing our new macro (for a small-*n* repeated measures design with replicates) to demonstrate how the macro listings and explanations in the appendices can enable readers to extend the range of designs in the book to include special problems of their own.

Appendix 1 gives useful tips for anyone not familiar with using random numbers and also offers help with other relevant skills that you may not have needed for ordinary statistical work. Appendices 2 and 3 list the macros with explanations for anyone contemplating more ambitious projects.

Acknowledgments

We want to thank the University of Dundee for support for this project, especially Trevor Harley, head of the Department of Psychology; Mark Bennett, who supported the appointment of one of us as honorary lecturer; and John Morris, whose technical support has always gone beyond the call of duty. We are also grateful to our friend and colleague Harry Staines who read some chapters, made useful comments, and gave us an example used in Chapter 7. Many readers have contacted us over the years with queries, and improvements in clarity are largely because you made us see the need for it! Among readers, we must mention Inna Tsirlin of York University in Canada, who prompted us to write a new macro and kindly allowed us to illustrate it with her example (which we have simplified a bit). Routledge/Taylor Francis reviewers Marie S. Hammond (Tennessee State University), Michele Ennis Soreth (Rowan University), Kimberly J. Vannest (Texas A & M University), and one anonymous reviewer made helpful suggestions, but any deficiencies remaining are our own. Andrea Zekus at Routledge/Taylor Francis helped us by always answering our questions about the production and so smoothed the process. Most of all we, are grateful to John Todman for many years of inspiration. This edition owes a great deal to him, not only for his work on the first edition but also for his vision and enthusiasm. Before his death in 2009, he said how much he wished he could work on a new edition that would be accessible to a wider audience.

Pat Dugard

Portia File

Jonathan Todman

chapter one

Single-case and small-n designs in context

Introduction

This book is intended to help researchers, students, and teachers in clinical, educational, and other areas involving human participants. Research in these areas is often aimed at testing the efficacy of a treatment or intervention in improving some measure of health or well-being. Psychologists seeking to understand human behavior also often test the effect of an intervention, treatment, or other experimental condition. There are well-established procedures for designing experiments where treatments or interventions can be randomly allocated to large numbers of participants who are representative of a well-defined population. We refer to such designs as *large-n* or *large-group designs*. Tests such as *t* tests and analysis of variance (ANOVA), known collectively as *parametric tests*, generally provide valid analyses of such designs provided some assumptions about the data are approximately met.

However, in much research involving people, the availability of individuals within specific categories is limited, making large-*n* studies impractical. It is no solution to increase the numbers available by defining the category broadly, because then the large differences among individuals within the broad category are likely to reduce drastically the power of the tests to detect any treatment effect. This is not the only reason why single-case and small-*n* designs may be used. They are also needed in exploratory research, for studying change over time, and to give a fine-grained focus on effectiveness in particular circumstances. In fact, single-case and small-*n* studies play a key role in the overall research strategy in the human sciences.

Levels of sophistication in single-case and small-n studies

Small-scale studies range in complexity from informal observation through formal case studies to formal observation of intervention effects. All these types of investigation have their place in the overall research effort, as we discuss in the next section, "Single-Case and Small-*n* Designs in the Research Process." Our purpose here is to convince you that, if you are considering a small-scale study, it is worth the effort of going beyond careful observation to full experimental design and analysis.

As an example, consider a neuropsychologist in a rehabilitation ward, helping patients who have suffered a traumatic brain injury. These patients often have very individual problems, so it sometimes takes creative imagination as well as knowledge and experience to suggest a treatment that may help. The neuropsychologist makes a suggestion for a particularly difficult case. The patient is keen to try something new, the treatment goes ahead, and all members of the ward team watch hopefully for progress. The patient too is eagerly watching for improvements. At the next case conference, everyone agrees that the new treatment has made some positive difference.

Where can the team take this from here? The evidence of their own eyes seems to show they have made some progress on a difficult case, yet it remains possible that in their enthusiasm to make a difference, they have seen changes where none exist. Alternatively, they may have witnessed real change that is a part of the natural course of the patient's condition and the treatment was irrelevant. It is possible to increase confidence in these results, but at some cost in terms of staff time, effort, and resources. The team may be tempted instead to spread the word about the apparent success so that others can research it further while they return to treating their patients.

But we want to convince clinicians and others that supporting their own observations with good experimental evidence is a realistic option for them. It is not true that the only way to provide convincing evidence of any effect is a large experiment with huge resources and a large staff followed by statistical analysis. It is also not true that statistical analysis always needs a large dataset. The key objective in designing an experiment is described next, and then we introduce the statistical tool that is the subject of this book.

Experimental design and internal validity

The key objective in any experimental design is the elimination of alternative explanations for any treatment effect observed. For instance, if cancer patients on the new drug live longer than those on the standard treatment, we want to know that the new drug is the explanation rather than some alternative such as the following: "The patients on the new drug were all treated by a specially dedicated team that gave emotional support as well, whereas the others attended the usual clinic where treatment was more impersonal." *Internal validity* is the term used for this elimination of alternative explanations. A good experimental design removes all threats to internal validity. (An experiment has *external validity* if the results can be applied to a wider population than those participating, and we discuss this in Chapters 3 and 6.)

An important tool in achieving internal validity is randomization. Notice that this is not at all the same as random sampling. Random sampling means choosing a sample from a well-defined population by using random numbers. Parametric tests assume the sample used for the experiment is obtained in this way, though in practice this is hardly ever true, and we discuss this fully in Chapter 6. Randomization refers to the method of allocating different treatments, conditions, or interventions. In large-n designs, treatments or interventions are randomly assigned to participants. Of course this is impossible in single-case studies, but it may be possible to randomly assign treatments to observation occasions. If we make a series of observations on a single case, or on a few cases, we can think of each as an *observation occasion*. If we make just one observation on a participant, then that too is an observation occasion. Randomly assigning treatments to participants is just one example of randomly assigning treatments to observation occasions.

Randomization tests: the tool we need

There are two reasons why we may not be able to apply the familiar parametric tests to the data when we have single-case or small-n designs, even if we do randomly allocate treatments to observation occasions. We did mention that there are several assumptions that need to be at least approximately true for the tests to be valid, and the smaller the number of observations, the harder it is to tell whether the assumptions are reasonable. One solution to uncertainty about the assumptions is to use nonparametric tests such as Mann-Whitney or Wilcoxon. These and other common nonparametric tests use ranks rather than actual observations, so some information is lost and the tests may lack sensitivity when applied to small groups. The other problem, especially relevant to single-case designs, is that parametric tests assume that the observations are independent. If we take a series of measurements on a single case, it is quite likely that if one measurement is high for some reason unrelated to the treatment, then the next measurement may also be a bit high. In other words, neighboring observations may be correlated and the observations are not independent. We discuss this more fully in Chapters 3 and 7.

The problems outlined in the previous paragraph do not apply to randomization tests. To use randomization tests, we do not need to make the parametric assumptions. Also for single-case designs, we need not assume the observations are independent, though as we shall see, large correlations among neighboring observations will reduce our chance of detecting a treatment effect. Randomization tests also do not rely on the unrealistic assumption of random sampling from a population. Thus, randomization tests provide us with the tools we need to analyze single-case and small-n studies, but we need to plan for them at the design stage, so designs and tests should be studied together, as in this book. Randomization tests can also be used for large-n studies, but well-known techniques already in use are fairly satisfactory and there is always resistance to change. However, we discuss their possible future role in Chapter 6.

Before proceeding to the study of randomization tests, how they work, and how to plan for them with suitable designs, we briefly review the important but often unconsidered part that small-scale studies play in the wider research process. This is the subject of the next section. We follow this with a short explanation of why, if randomization tests are so useful, they are so little known. Finally, we end this chapter with some notes on how you might use the book.

Single-case and small-n designs in the research process

The scientific method of gaining new knowledge and understanding imposes similar structures and constraints on researchers in most areas of enquiry. We use the example of clinical research to show how single-case and small-n studies fit into the wider picture of the research effort.

A model of the clinical research process

In clinical research, as in other areas, the randomized controlled trial (RCT) is seen as the gold standard for research. This reputation is deserved and is an important achievement of 20th-century science, but it does not provide what is needed for every study or every stage in the research process. In particular, the early stages of developing a new idea do not lend themselves to large experiments. Also, in clinical work, although a well-run RCT can do a great job of answering questions about the average improvement due to an intervention, a clinician usually wants to know whether it works for a particular patient.

Robey (2004) proposed a hierarchical model (Table 1.1) for the whole clinical research process, in which single-case and small-n designs appear in the first two phases and again in the fourth phase. As can be seen, in this model there is a place for RCTs, single-case and small-n designs, and qualitative, meta-analytic, and cost-effectiveness studies. A similar structure, beginning with identification of a promising idea, through small

Table 1.1 Robey's Model of the Clinical Research Process

Phase	Purpose	Methods
I	Identifying a therapeutic effect and estimating its magnitude	Exploratory qualitative, single-case, and small-group designs
II	Exploring the dimensions of the therapeutic effect and preparing for a clinical trial	Experimental single-case and small-group studies, and reliability and validity studies
III	Clinical trial to test efficacy	RCT, independent replication
IV	Field research to test effectiveness in target population, subpopulations, variations in service delivery, and variants of protocol	Meta-analyses, and experimental single-case and small-group studies
V	Who benefits, and at what cost?	Cost-effectiveness investigations

and then large studies to replication and finally cost-effectiveness studies, could be identified in other research areas. To get the best results, we need to use all these methods in their proper place.

As can be seen in the above model, there are times when single-case and small-*n* studies are appropriate and times when they are not. Exploratory studies and some individual clinical studies fall into Phase I and II of Robey's model. Studying effects under different conditions would be part of Phase IV. However, the use of RCTs in Phase III of Robey's model is wholly appropriate and small-*n* designs are unlikely to add much at this stage. There is now a huge body of knowledge about the best ways to design, manage, and analyze large RCTs and other experiments with large samples. In contrast, and despite the apparent usefulness outlined in Robey's model, single-case and small-*n* designs have received far less attention. This book is a contribution to extending the knowledge of how best to use experimental opportunities with much smaller groups.

Consider the place of single-case and small-*n* research in each of the areas identified by Robey: exploratory studies, individual clinical studies, and studying effects under different conditions.

Exploratory studies

At some stage in the research process we must find an idea worth testing, and such an idea may come about by keeping an eye open for surprise developments and possible causes. When an observant scientist with a sense of curiosity notices an anomaly in research data or clinical experience and chooses not to ignore it, there is the possibility that a new and good idea will be born. Such new ideas may just as easily come from an experienced practitioner or from a young newcomer who brings a fresh perspective and is too inexperienced to have preconceived ideas. All practicing scientists need to use their senses and listen to their intuition, but it takes some confidence and judgment to know when to pursue an unusual observation.

As a first step, investigating a single case or a very small group may be possible with quite modest resources, and this may clarify the idea and suggest what form a larger study should take. Alternatively several small-group studies may be used to lay out the directions for future work or to prepare for a large experiment such as a major clinical trial.

Individual clinical studies

To find out about the effectiveness of an intervention for an individual patient, we have to collect data from that individual. We need a single-case design. At this level of individual studies, it is clinicians or others working with individual patients or clients who need to be able to choose, implement, and analyze results from a single-case design. They are the ones who see the details, who can see exactly what they need to find out, and who know which patients may be able to provide the answers.

Many clinicians must also try to help patients whose condition is very unusual, or for which no effective treatment has been reported. In such cases it may be possible to adapt an intervention that has helped those with a related problem, and, if the patient is willing to try something new, then progress may be made that will help others as well.

Studying effects under different conditions

Once the average or general effects are understood, it may be necessary to investigate the effects of varying the circumstances, conditions, or method of delivery on whatever we are studying. Small-*n* or even single-case studies may again have a part to play in this process. If we are studying a treatment or intervention for patients or clients, then the great variety among individuals makes it likely that some will benefit much more than others. Studying small subgroups or individual cases is the best way to tease out the details of how to administer the treatment in different circumstances, or how to decide whether it will help in particular cases.

Whether we are asking GPs to apply the results of clinical drug trials or taking the results from educational trials in tightly controlled environments to classroom practice, we are assuming that what was observed in large experiments in carefully controlled conditions will also be found in real-world application, so we should certainly do everything possible to find out how changes in circumstances might affect results. Some of this work can be done by including studies of small subgroups as part of the main investigation, but clinicians or others responsible for applying the findings can also contribute their own observations on single cases or small groups. Such observations, when carefully recorded and shared, greatly add to the pool of knowledge.

Each of these components of the whole research agenda has a clear role for single-case and small-*n* studies. However, whether for historical, educational, or practical reasons, designs with small numbers of participants have been somewhat sidelined over the years. With randomization tests now coming of age, perhaps it is time for a more balanced view of research that puts every design in its proper place.

Randomization tests' time has come

If randomization tests are so useful, why are they not more widely known? There are several reasons that we discuss in Chapter 2, but for now we just mention the main one, which is historical. The development of computing lagged behind the need for statistical methods in research. Randomization tests were first suggested more than 80 years ago, but their use was very limited until fast computing became generally available in the last quarter of the 20th century. By then, researchers had become accustomed to a different approach to statistics, and research methods courses were focused on those techniques that had become familiar. Powerful statistical software, increasingly used by any serious researcher, did not include randomization tests.

A seminal work by Eugene Edgington in 1980 (now in its fourth edition [2007], coauthored with Patrick Onghena) contained Fortran programs to make randomization tests more readily available, but even this did not result in their widespread use. With the first edition of this book (2001), we tried to make these unfamiliar methods more accessible with an introductory account and the means to perform the tests in a familiar software environment (SPSS, Excel, or Minitab). In this edition we have given much fuller explanations and many more examples, and we hope many more potential users will see how they can be applied in their own work.

Using this book

This book is an introductory treatment of a subject not covered in most research methods courses. Researchers and students new to the area will find all they need to start applying randomization designs and tests to their own investigations. However, although this is an introductory text, for those encountering the ideas for the first time it does not make easy reading. Most people will need several attempts before they feel really confident with the material, especially Chapters 2 and 4. For anyone who finds their needs outstripping the tools demonstrated here, we provide advice in Chapter 8 about where to find more advanced techniques.

We provide the tools to design and analyze experiments with one or a few cases. You can analyze your own data using our macros in SPSS or Excel. We provide the macros and full instructions in their use. The macros and example data are on the book Web site (http://www.researchmethodsarena.com/9780415886932). They form a central feature of the book, providing as they do the opportunity to implement randomization tests in a familiar software environment, but much of the text is devoted to explaining how randomization tests work and how to use them.

We would urge everyone unfamiliar with randomization tests to study Chapter 2, which contains explanations of the key ideas and introductory examples for some of the designs. Chapter 3 outlines the conditions in which each of the randomization designs can be used, and you would use this to decide on an appropriate design for your own problem. Chapter 4 explains the details of implementing each of the designs. When you finish Chapter 3, you should have a good idea of which designs may be suitable for any small sample problem you have, though when you get down to the details in Chapter 4 you may find you have to revise your plan. You may also need to reread relevant sections of Chapter 2 as you consider which design is best for a particular problem. Going through the generalities to identify a candidate design, then attempting to implement it using the detailed instructions in Chapter 4, and then needing to return to the generalities, comprise an iterative process you may need to go through several times, especially if you are not a very experienced researcher.

Once you have chosen your design and understood how to implement it, then you can move on to Chapter 5, which demonstrates the analysis for each design. The macros in SPSS and Excel perform the analyses, and in case you haven't used macros before, we show you how at the beginning of Appendix 2 (SPSS) and Appendix 3 (Excel). Then you can easily take the macro you want from the Web site and apply it to your own data using the instructions in Chapter 4 (and, if you need help running the macro, at the start of the appendix for your chosen package). Note that much of the material in Appendices 2 and 3 is only needed by advanced users as described in Chapter 8.

Chapters 3 to 5 form the "how to do it" guide to randomization designs and tests, but even if your main interest is practical, we encourage you to read on, and if you are studying research methods, then Chapters 6 and 7 are essential reading. In Chapter 6 we discuss how randomization tests free the experimenter from the necessity of pretending that their cases can be regarded as if they formed a random sample, a fiction that underpins most statistical analyses. We show the effect of the random-sampling fiction on external validity and discuss how external validity is actually achieved for both randomization and more traditional designs. Also in Chapter 6 we show how randomization increases confidence in internal validity, especially when used in *phase designs*. Finally, in this chapter we consider cases where we might gain some information from performing a randomization test even where correct randomization was not performed.

Chapter 7 is where we consider the power of randomization tests, and also some ways in which power may be enhanced. Much of this advice is just best practice for any experimenter, but it may be particularly important for small-scale work. The phase designs often have rather low power, and if you plan to use one of these you should certainly read this chapter.

Chapter 8 is for those who want to go further than this introductory treatment. In it we list some other sources of software for performing randomization tests, including some for many designs we have not described. There is also some recommended further reading. If you want to write macros in SPSS or Excel for other designs, we offer some general advice and also demonstrate with an example how you might reuse and adapt some of the code from our macros.

We list the macros (in Appendices 2 and 3) with explanations for the benefit of anyone who wants to go further and start writing their own macros for other designs. Until you want to do this, the only parts of these appendices you need are the introductory sections with instructions for running the macros. To use the macros with your own data we recommend taking them from the book Web site, where they are listed without the added explanations.

We have assumed a basic knowledge of statistics: In particular we do not explain the terms null hypothesis, alternative hypothesis, *t* test, analysis of variance (ANOVA), *F*, residual sum of squares (RSS), one-tailed test, two-tailed test, correlation, and sum of products. We use the standard notation for means and sums. A little knowledge of non-parametric tests will be useful. We do not provide an introduction to SPSS or Excel, and we assume you know how to set up a datasheet in your chosen package and perform simple manipulations. If you get to the stage of wanting to write your own macros (we guess this will be a minority of our readers), you will need some knowledge of the SPSS matrix language (look up matrix language in the help index) or, for Excel, Visual Basic. Many books give an introduction to Visual Basic for Excel.

We have not assumed any knowledge of randomization tests: We aim to make these accessible for anyone starting from the position described in the previous paragraph. We do not assume you know how to find a random number, arrange things in random order, or otherwise use the random number facilities of SPSS or Excel. These are basic skills for someone wanting to use randomization designs, and we have collected instructions in Appendix 1 so that we do not need to interrupt the flow of exposition with these details. We often draw your attention to Appendix 1 when we make use of these skills, but you can always leave finding out about them until later, so that you can concentrate on the design.

We have provided a glossary. When a technical term is used for the first time it is italicized, and you will find a brief definition in the glossary. We also use italics sometimes for emphasis.

Chapters 2 to 7 have some exercises for the reader. You can find solutions on the book Web site (http://www.researchmethodsarena. com/9780415886932), but we urge you to try them yourself. The questions are designed to get you to think about things in a slightly different way or to notice something in the text that you may not have considered. The preceding text always contains what you need to find the answers, and if trying the questions gets you to reread parts of it, this will help to consolidate your understanding.

All the examples throughout the book demonstrate the designs in realistic situations. The data are fabricated so that the important points are clearly made. When working with real data, we often have to consider complicating features, but when learning about unfamiliar techniques for the first time, we need to avoid distraction. So our data, fabricated for the purpose, allow us to tackle issues one at a time.

chapter two

Understanding randomization tests

An introductory example: testing for extrasensory perception (ESP)

The fundamental problem of statistical inference is the same as that facing a jury in a court of law: How should the evidence be weighed? In science, just as in the law courts, the cases where the truth is clear and obvious are rather rare. Usually many discrepancies of unknown importance obscure the facts. In this book we shall explore one of the approaches developed to uncover the truth that may not be obvious from experimental data. Scientists working with animals and plants, and even more so with humans, have to accept that however hard they try to compare like with like, there are differences among individuals and among observation occasions that may affect the measurements. Only in the 20th century did statisticians begin to systematically investigate ways to assess the evidence provided by data that included such variation. The familiar methods of hypothesis testing are the most widely used results of these researches. But another approach, tried out early on but shelved for lack of computing power, led to the randomization tests that are the subject of this book. Now that fast computing is available to everyone, the uses of these tests can be explored.

We will begin with an example. Suppose someone strongly believes she has extrasensory perception (ESP) and can tell when she is being covertly watched. We would like to do an experiment designed to test the claim. More specifically, we would like to test the hypothesis that she could discriminate between occasions when an experimenter is observing her and occasions when he is not. She will sit alone in a room, where the experimenter can view her though a closed-circuit television (CCTV) camera or where he can look away and not view her. There will be eight test periods of one minute, four when the experimenter will be watching her (V) and four when he will not (N). At the end of each test period, she must respond by writing a V if she thinks she is being watched and an N if she thinks she is not. Her answer will be a list of her eight V and N

Table 2.1 Obtaining an Arrangement of Four Vs and Four Ns

Step	Result	Arrangement So Far	Items Left
1	Tail	N	VVVVNNN
2	Head	NV	VVVNNN
3	Head	NVV	VVNNN
4	Tail	NVVN	VVNN
5	Head	NVVNV	VNN
6	Head	NVVNVV	NN
7		NVVNVVNN	

responses. Even if she does not have ESP and is only guessing, she will probably have some correct responses. But how do we know if she can really tell the difference? Suppose she got them all correct: How likely would that be if she was just guessing?

Because we need to present our ESP claimant with the Vs and Ns in random order for our experiment, let's look first at how one possible arrangement of the Vs and Ns could be obtained by tossing a coin. We start with the eight items, VVVVNNNN, and we must choose one for each testing occasion. After selecting an item, we cannot use it again. Essentially, we have eight blank spaces that we want to fill with eight items. Once all the Vs or all the Ns are used, the remaining spaces are filled by the remaining letters. The order that these items fall in constitutes one arrangement. Let's say we choose V when we throw a head. Table 2.1 shows an example of the process. We could also obtain a random ordering of four Vs and four Ns as described in Appendix 1.

To find out how likely it is that our ESP claimant could get all correct answers by guessing, we need to know how many possible arrangements of four Vs and four Ns there are. The next section shows how to find out.

Calculating the number of possible arrangements

Think first of how many ways there are to arrange 8 different items in order. There are 8 items to choose for the first item, then only 7 items left to choose for the second, so 8*7 ways to choose the first two items. Now there are 6 items to choose for the third item, 5 items to choose for the fourth, and so on until there is only one choice for the last item. So there are 8*7*6*5*4*3*2*1 ways to arrange 8 different items in order. We write this as 8!, called 8 factorial, and it's a large number (40,320).

But now suppose four of the items are identical, so if they are rearranged among themselves we won't notice. To see this, suppose we have four different items, V_1, V_2, V_3, V_4 and four identical items, N, N, N, and

N. An arrangement such as $V_1NNV_2V_3NV_4N$ looks exactly the same however you rearrange the Ns among themselves. There are 4! or 4*3*2*1 or 24 ways to rearrange the four Ns among themselves. So if we could tell the Ns apart, we would have 24 different arrangements with the Vs in these positions, but instead we have only one. This will apply wherever the Vs are, so of our 8! arrangements, only 8!/4! (or 1,680) will look different. Now if the other four items are also identical (but different from the first four), only 8!/(4!4!), or 70, will look different. So this is how many different answers our ESP claimant could give us.

Another word often used for arrangements of items such as we have been discussing is *permutations*. So we could say there are 70 permutations of eight objects, four each of two kinds. In general, there are N! ways to arrange N different items. If A of them are identical, then there are only N!/A! different permutations. If another B of them are identical but different from the As, then we have only N!/(A!B!) different permutations. If another C are identical but different from the As and Bs, there are only N!/(A!B!C!) different permutations, and so on.

Performing the experiment

So for our experiment, we choose one of the 70 permutations of four Vs and four Ns at random and the observer carries out the selected sequence of viewing and not viewing her. She knows there are four of each, and she writes down what she thinks is the correct sequence, which will look something like VVNVVNNN. The null hypothesis is that actually she can't tell whether she is being observed or not, and if this is the case, her list of Vs and Ns bears no relation to reality—it's just one of the 70 possible arrangements of four Vs and four Ns chosen at random. If every V and N in her sequence is correct, then this clearly supports her case as it would be a very lucky guess to get the right one out of 70 arrangements.

If we are doing an ordinary hypothesis test, we say the result is significant at the 5% level if the probability that it occurs at random when the null hypothesis is true is less than 5%. One chance in 70 is only 1.4%, which is less than 5%, so if our ESP claimant gets them all right, we reject the null hypothesis (that she cannot tell when she is being covertly watched) at the 5% level. The evidence supports her claim that she can tell when she is being watched.

The ESP experiment is an example of a randomization design that is analogous to designs for use with analysis of variance (ANOVA). In the next section, we describe three groups of randomization tests: analogies to ANOVA like the ESP example, phase designs where measurements are taken before and after an intervention, and designs to investigate order effects. All of the designs described in this book belong to one of these groups.

Classes of randomization tests
Analogs of ANOVA

We used the ESP experiment as our introductory example because the experimental setup is one of the simplest experimental designs. It is a special case of a one-way ANOVA with just two treatments or experimental conditions. Here our two experimental conditions are "being watched" (V) and "not being watched" (N). If the ANOVA design has only two conditions, either a *t* test or the usual *F* test can be applied.

Our eight test periods are the observation occasions, and four each of V and N are randomly assigned to them. Whether we are setting up a *t* test or a randomization test, we can achieve the random assignment in several ways. We could list the 70 possible arrangements and choose one at random; we could toss a coin and assign V for a head and N for a tail until we have used all four of one condition, then assign the rest to the other (as in Table 2.1); or we could arrange V, V, V, V, N, N, N, and N in random order as shown in Appendix 1.

For a *t* test, we would calculate the *t* from a measurement made on the Vs and the Ns and then compare the *t* with its table of probabilities to see whether the obtained *t* value would have a less than 5% chance of occurring if the null hypothesis is true. In our ESP example, we have a very simple measurement: We just record whether the V or N is correct for each test period. Then we compare the number correct with all the other possible arrangements of Vs and Ns. We shall consider several designs for randomization tests that have experimental setups like analysis of variance (or *t* tests if there are only two conditions). We refer to this group of designs as analogs of ANOVA.

Phase designs

Another important class of randomization tests consists of the *phase designs*. The simplest phase design takes a single individual or "case" and observes or takes a measurement on a series of occasions. The measurement can be physiological (blood pressure), psychological (anxiety level), or behavioral (a count of aggressive interactions). After the first few observations, there is an intervention (usually some treatment or training), and then the rest of the observations (called intervention observations) are taken. The observations before the intervention form the *baseline phase* (A), and those taken from the intervention onward form the *intervention phase* (B). This is an AB design.

The intervention may be a drug or therapy where any effect will be maintained only as long as the participant continues to receive it, or a once-only intervention, such as some training, that is expected to have a long-lasting effect. Whether the intervention is a one-off occurrence such as a training session or surgical procedure, or the start of continuing treatment such as a daily drug dose, all the observations from the intervention onward are called the intervention phase.

Whatever measurement we make will be likely to show some intrinsic variability from one measurement occasion to the next. For example, blood pressure is likely to be different each time we measure it even when we are not doing anything deliberately that might influence it. This natural variability can obscure any effect that the intervention has, and part of the reason for making a series of observations both before and after the intervention is to give a reasonable chance of seeing any effect of the intervention in spite of the variability.

A critical judgment when designing the study will be deciding how many observation occasions are required. First, we will wish to gain an estimate of baseline and intervention levels in order to see if there is a before–after difference. Second, for a phase design to qualify as a randomization design, the intervention point must be chosen at random from a set of possible observation occasions. For this to be possible, we need more observation occasions than we would need just to get a good estimate of the baseline and intervention levels.

Suppose we are taking a measurement and we will use the mean of each phase as our indicator of the baseline and intervention levels. If we need at least five observations in each phase to get a good estimate of the means, then to set up a randomization test we need more than 10 observation occasions (probably a lot more). If we have 15 possible observation occasions, then we could choose the intervention point at random from those possible, which would be observations 6, 7, 8, 9, 10, or 11 as shown in Table 2.2.

If the intervention is introduced at observation 11, we have just five occasions left to observe the intervention phase. If the intervention is introduced at observations 6, we have just five occasions before that to observe the baseline phase. Any point in between will satisfy the constraint of at least five observations for each phase.

Table 2.2 An AB Design With 15 Observations, at Least 5 in Each Phase

Intervention point	Baseline phase	*n* for Baseline	Intervention phase	*n* for Intervention
6	1–5	5	6–15	10
7	1–6	6	7–15	9
8	1–7	7	8–15	8
9	1–8	8	9–15	7
10	1–9	9	10–15	6
11	1–10	10	11–15	5

Phase designs can be extended to include more than one case, though usually there will be only a small number. These are called *multiple baseline phase designs*. Phase designs can also be extended to include a *reversal* or *withdrawal phase* if the intervention is a treatment that can be withdrawn. However, withdrawal may not be possible for practical or ethical reasons. If a withdrawal phase is included, we have an ABA design. ABA designs can also be used with more than one case.

Order effects

We shall also discuss a small group of designs that examine order effects, though, as we shall see, a purist might reject some of them on the grounds that the randomization process may be incomplete. Sometimes an observer may be able to arrange effects in order even if he or she is unable to assign values. For instance, a participant may be able to arrange a small set of stimuli in order of painfulness, without being able to assign a pain level to a place on a scale. We may want to know whether the ordering of a set of stimuli is related to another ordering such as the amount of information about the stimuli given to the participant.

We may be able to manage only a *partial ordering*, as when an interviewer judges that two of the candidates are excellent, three others could do the job, and one is hopeless. Here the six candidates have been partially ordered into three categories, but the interviewer is unable to order those within the first two categories. We can use the test with partial orderings as well.

So we have three classes of randomization tests to explore: analogs of ANOVA, phase designs, and order effects.

Hypothesis tests for randomization designs

The first requirement for any of our familiar hypothesis tests is a *test statistic* such as t, F, or χ^2. This may be an unfamiliar way to think of them, but each is a summary of our data designed to expose the particular feature we are testing. Take the t, for instance, which is the test statistic for deciding whether two groups have the same mean. The t we calculate from the data has the difference between our two sample means as the numerator. The denominator is an estimate of variability based on pooled data from both samples. So t is large if the difference between sample means is large compared to the variability within the observations.

To perform one of the usual hypothesis tests, we compare the test statistic such as t or F with a table of probabilities (or else a package such as SPSS gives us the probability along with the test statistic). Randomization tests use a different approach, where the unused possible randomizations are the basis of the comparison. To show you how this works, we look again at the ESP experiment, and then at some examples from each group of randomization designs.

We chose at random one of the 70 possible arrangements of four Vs and four Ns to present to our ESP claimant, she made a list of four Vs and four Ns, and we saw how many she got correct. If she got them all right, then either she chose the correct arrangement from the list of 70 by chance (probability 1/70), or she really can tell the difference. So, "all correct" is a result significant at the 5% level.

But suppose she gets most but not all of them right; how do we assess the evidence then? Suppose the actual arrangement was VVNVNNVN, but she wrote down VVNVVNNN, so her score was six correct. How many of the other arrangements have at least six correct? A moment's reflection tells you the number correct has to be 0, 2, 4, 6, or 8 because she knows there are four of each and if one is placed incorrectly another must be also. Here are a few other arrangements with six of their Vs and Ns in the same place as the actual arrangement we gave to our ESP claimant, with the incorrect ones in italic.

VVN*NN*VVN
V*N*VVNNVN
VN*N*VN*V*VN
*N*VVVNNVN

Though tedious, it is possible in this case to list by hand all the 70 arrangements and for each one count the number of Vs and Ns that are correct compared with the arrangement actually used. These counts form the *reference set*. There are 16 with six correct, including the one our claimant wrote down, and we showed you some of them above. If she can't really tell the difference between V and N, she could have chosen one of these 16 or the one with all correct out of the 70 just by chance with a probability of 17/70, or 24%. This is not small enough for us to reject the null hypothesis. In fact, in this experiment, unless she gets all eight correct, we won't believe her claim to know the difference.

Five steps to devising a randomization test

This example illustrates the steps in devising a randomization test. (The calculations in steps 3 and 4 will be done by a macro.)

   1. State the hypotheses. (Our null hypothesis [H_0] is that our claimant cannot tell when she is being watched. Our alternative [or experimental] hypothesis [H_1] is that she can tell.)

2. Choose at random an arrangement from a list of suitable ones (we had 70 arrangements of four Vs and four Ns). The full list of suitable arrangements will be used to obtain the reference set (step 4).
3. Calculate a test statistic from the experiment (we counted the number of test periods correctly identified as V or N).
4. Calculate the same test statistic for all the unused arrangements (we counted the number correct for each of the other 69 arrangements). This is the reference set.
5. Compare the actual statistic from the experiment with those from the unused arrangements (the reference set). What is the percentage at least as extreme as our actual one? This percentage gives the probability of obtaining a result at least as extreme as ours by chance.

Step 2 can often be performed in several different ways, and sometimes we show you more than one. It is important to note that the method of randomization is part of the design, and if you intend to use our macros, the randomization must be performed in a way consistent with the design. Also care must be taken that whatever method is used for step 2, the same method is used for identifying the arrangements used in step 4. We expand on this point in Chapter 4, where we show how to implement the designs covered in the book, but for this chapter just concentrate on following the steps through the example designs.

As you read these examples, you may wonder how you would do the calculations for step 4. In fact, all calculations will be done by the macros, so just concentrate on following the method.

Analogs of ANOVA: a one-way design for a single case

Step 1: The example problem with the hypotheses

We extend the ESP example to a case where we have three experimental conditions. Suppose we want to compare different methods of pain control for a patient with arthritis. The study can run for 7 weeks, and in each week we will use one of the methods of pain control (the drug paracetamol, hypnosis, and acupuncture). So the conditions are

- Level 1: Paracetamol
- Level 2: Hypnosis
- Level 3: Acupuncture

Three of the weeks will be assigned to paracetamol, with 2 weeks each for the other treatments, in random order. Notice that we do not need to have equal numbers of observations for the experimental conditions. Our hypotheses are

H_0: The three pain control methods are equally effective.
H_1: The three pain control methods are not equally effective.

Step 2: Choose a random arrangement from those suitable

There are 7! ways to assign seven different treatments to weeks, but if three of them are the same (the drug), there are only 7!/3! arrangements that are distinct. If two of the remaining four are the same (hypnosis), there are 7!/(3!2!) distinct arrangements; and if the last two are also the same (acupuncture), we have 7!/(3!2!2!) or 210 distinct arrangements. Either we can list these and choose one at random for the experiment, or we can achieve the same result as follows. We code the treatments 1 (paracetamol), 2 (hypnosis), and 3 (acupuncture). Because we want to use 3 weeks for the drug and 2 each for the other treatments, arrange 1, 1, 1, 2, 2, 3, and 3 in random order (Appendix 1 shows how to do this). Apply the treatments to the weeks in the random order we obtain.

Step 3: Choose a test statistic

The patient will keep a pain diary from which a score will be derived for each week. The null hypothesis is that all the methods are equally effective for controlling the pain. Unlike in the ESP experiment, it is not obvious what we should use as our test statistic. If we had only two treatments, we could use the difference between mean scores, but we need a statistic to compare three. Clearly the greater the differences are among the three treatment mean scores, relative to the variability of the scores within each treatment, the stronger is the evidence against the null hypothesis. If you have used ANOVA, you will know that Fisher's F is a measure of this: The bigger the F, the greater the differences among treatment means relative to the variability within treatment groups. (If you are not familiar with ANOVA and F, you can either just accept that F is a suitable test statistic or learn more about it in almost any statistical textbook, such as Howell [2010] or Dugard, Todman, & Staines [2010].) We can calculate the value of F (or let our macro do it) for our actual data in exactly the same way as we would for an ANOVA, and then use this statistic for our randomization test.

Step 4: Calculate the test statistic for all unused arrangements

Now suppose the null hypothesis is true: In this case, the treatment label (drug, hypnosis, or acupuncture) associated with each week is quite

Table 2.3 Actual F and One From the Reference Set

Week	Pain score	Actual treatment	Rearrangement
1	5	2	3
2	7	2	3
3	5	3	2
4	2	1	1
5	6	3	1
6	4	1	1
7	3	1	2
		$\bar{x}_1 = 3.0, \bar{x}_2 = 6.0, \bar{x}_3 = 5.5$	$\bar{x}_1 = 4.0, \bar{x}_2 = 4.0, \bar{x}_3 = 6.0$
		$F = 5.873$	$F = 0.952$

arbitrary. We could rearrange the labels in any way we like, and any difference in our calculated F will just be due to random variation. This is the key to the randomization test. Table 2.3 shows an example, with the actual F from the experiment and one of the values obtained by rearranging the treatment labels. Rearrange the labels in all the 210 ways, and calculate F for each of them. This is the reference set. The macros do the calculations for you, so you do not have to know how to do this in detail.

Step 5: Compare the actual statistic with those from the unused arrangements

Now see where the F for the actual arrangement used in our experiment falls in the reference set. If the null hypothesis is not true, and there are differences among the treatments, the F from the actual experiment should be larger than those obtained by randomly rearranging the treatment labels. Is it the largest? In the top three or the top 10? With 210 possible arrangements, if the actual one used gives an F in the top 10 (4.8%), we would have a result significant at the 5% level.

Analogs of ANOVA: a single-case 2*2 factorial design

Step 1: The example problem with the hypotheses

Suppose now that we wish to test whether a disruptive child behaves better in the classroom if accompanied by a carer. This is obviously an expensive solution, so evidence for effectiveness is needed. There is already some suggestion that the child may be more troublesome in the afternoon than the morning. There are two factors each with two levels. Factor 1 is carer present (C, level 1) or not (U, level 2). Factor 2 is morning (M, level 1) or afternoon (A, level 2). The four conditions will be

- CM: Carer present for a morning session
- CA: Carer present for an afternoon session
- UM: Carer absent for a morning session
- UA: Carer absent for an afternoon session

There is a null and alternative hypothesis for each factor. For factor 1, we have

H_0: The presence or absence of the carer does not affect disruptiveness.
H_1: The presence of the carer reduces disruptiveness.

And for factor 2:

H_0: The time of day (morning or afternoon) does not affect disruptiveness.
H_1: There is less disruption in the morning than the afternoon.

Step 2: Choose a random arrangement from those suitable
We will allow 12 days for the study, using either the morning or the afternoon of each day, to give us three observations for each of the four conditions, and we will apply them in random order to our 12 days. We can achieve the randomization easily. Number the conditions from 1 to 4 (e.g., CM is 1, CA is 2, UM is 3, and UA is 4), then arrange 1, 1, 1, 2, 2, 2, 3, 3, 3, 4, 4, and 4 in random order (Appendix 1 shows how). Apply the conditions to the 12 days in the random order obtained.

Step 3: Choose a test statistic
At each observation session, the teacher will be videoed and an independent assessor will count the occasions when she has to deal with disruption from the child. These counts will be our data. Our primary interest is in whether the presence of the carer reduces disruption, and we begin by looking first at the *main effect* of presence or absence of the carer. The test statistic would be the difference between means for the six U sessions and the six C sessions. If the carer makes no difference, then the labels C and U are arbitrary, and if they are rearranged over the 12 sessions, the only difference made in the test statistic will be due to random variation.

Step 4: Calculate the test statistic for all unused arrangements
The rearrangements must conform to the conditions of the experiment as set out in step 2, so the three Us and three Cs can be rearranged over the six morning sessions, and similarly over the six afternoon sessions. There are 6!/(3!3!) or 20 ways to rearrange the Us and Cs over the mornings and 20

Table 2.4 Actual Mean Difference and One From the Reference Set

Day	Count	Actual condition	Rearrangement
1	13	UA	UA
2	10	UA	CA
3	5	CA	CA
4	2	CA	UA
5	3	CM	UM
6	12	UM	CM
7	4	CA	UA
8	7	CM	CM
9	9	UM	CM
10	11	UA	CA
11	4	CM	UM
12	5	UM	UM
		$\overline{C} = 4.2, \overline{U} = 10.0, \overline{U} - \overline{C} = 5.8$	$\overline{C} = 9.0, \overline{U} = 5.2, \overline{U} - \overline{C} = -3.8$

ways to rearrange them over the afternoons. Because any morning arrangement can be paired with any afternoon arrangement, we have 20*20 or 400 arrangements in the reference set. This is the key to the randomization test. If our result is the top 20 (5%), we would have a result significant at the 5% level (using a one-tailed test). The macro will do the calculations.

Table 2.4 shows an example with the mean difference from the actual experiment and one rearrangement from the reference set.

Step 5: Compare the actual statistic with those from the unused arrangements

Once we have all the test statistics calculated from the unused rearrangements, look to see whether our actual one from the experiment is in the top 20 (5% of 400). If it is, the evidence supports the alternative hypothesis that the presence of the carer reduces disruptive behavior.

But the effect may not be the same in the morning and the afternoon, so we may wish to look at the *simple effects*. Our most direct approach to this is to look at the mornings and afternoons separately. This would correspond to looking at the simple effects from a two-factor ANOVA. We will go through the process for the simple effect of factor 1 (carer) in the morning.

Step 1

H_0: The presence or absence of the carer does not affect disruptiveness in the morning.

H_1: The presence of the carer reduces disruptiveness in the morning.

Step 2
This is already done.

Step 3
An obvious test statistic is the mean count for the three mornings without the carer minus the mean count for the three mornings with the carer.

Step 4
If the null hypothesis is true, and the presence of the carer makes no difference to the number of disruptions in morning sessions, then U and C are just arbitrary labels. So we can reassign them randomly to the six morning observations and recalculate the difference between means, and the result will differ from our actual one only because of the random variation among morning sessions. This is the key to the randomization test.

For the data in Table 2.4, for mornings we have $\overline{C} = 4.7$, $\overline{U} = 8.7$, and $\overline{U} - \overline{C} = 4.0$ in the actual experiment, and $\overline{C} = 9.3$, $\overline{U} = 4.0$, and $\overline{U} - \overline{C} = -5.3$ for one of the rearrangements.

There are $6!/(3!3!)$ or 20 ways to arrange three Us and three Cs over the 6 mornings, so we calculate the difference between the U and C means for each unused arrangement to get the reference set.

Step 5
If our actual result is bigger than any other in the reference set, then it is just significant at the 5% level.

We can repeat this process for afternoon sessions, and this should enable us to make a decision on whether to arrange for the carer to be present in the mornings, the afternoons, or both. If we are also interested in any possible difference between morning and afternoon sessions, we could first look at the main effect by rearranging the M and A labels across the 12 sessions, just as we rearranged the U and C labels to get the main effect of the carer. We could also look at the simple effects of M and A within the U sessions and within the C sessions. Note that there is no randomization test for interaction effects. Edgington and Onghena (2007) explained why this is so (and see "Further Reading" at the end of Chapter 8).

Phase designs: a single-case AB design

As we noted earlier, a phase design is useful when we wish to test whether the introduction of an intervention has an effect on our measurements. Now we take you through an example.

Step 1: The example problem with the hypotheses

A multiple sclerosis (MS) patient is willing to try out an intensive physiotherapy program that may improve her mobility. So we can use an AB phase design with a baseline phase (A) before an intervention phase (B).

To apply a randomization test to the AB design, we must choose the intervention point at random, so we need a set of points to choose from, any of which would be suitable. With our MS patient, her condition has changed little for a long time, and it will make no difference if the intervention is delayed by some weeks.

An independent physiotherapist, who will not know when we intervene with the intensive program, will assess our patient's mobility every week for 30 weeks. Between two of these assessments will be the intervention, which if effective will increase the patient's mobility score. The hypotheses are

H_0: The intensive physiotherapy will not affect mobility.
H_1: The intensive physiotherapy will improve mobility.

Step 2: Choose a random arrangement from those suitable

Because MS patients have good and bad days, we need at least five assessments in each of the two phases to get a good estimate of mobility in each phase. Then the intervention could be before

- Week 6 (weeks 1–5 for baseline and 6–30 for intervention)
- Week 7 (weeks 1–6 for baseline and 7–30 for intervention)
- Week 8 (weeks 1–7 for baseline and 8–30 for intervention)

... And so on up to

- Week 25 (weeks 1–24 for baseline and 25–30 for intervention)
- Week 26 (weeks 1–25 for baseline and 26–30 for intervention)

Suppose week 13 is randomly chosen from this list of possibilities. (Look at Appendix 1 if you are not sure how to choose a random number from within a range.)

Step 3: Choose a test statistic

Our test statistic would be the difference between the mean score for observations 13 to 30 (the intervention mean) and the mean score for the first 12 observations (the baseline mean). But how do we test for significance?

Table 2.5 Baseline and Intervention Means for Actual
and Two Reference Set Divisions

Divide at	Baseline (A)	Intervention (B)	Means
Week 13 (actual)	6, 8, 7, 7, 4, 4, 7, 11, 8, 7, 7, 6	12, 9, 9, 6, 8, 12, 12, 11, 9, 6, 14, 11, 10, 12, 9, 12, 11, 8	$\bar{x}_A = 6.8, \bar{x}_B = 10.1$ $\bar{x}_B - \bar{x}_A = 3.3$
Week 12	6, 8, 7, 7, 4, 4, 7, 11, 8, 7, 7,	6, 12, 9, 9, 6, 8, 12, 12, 11, 9, 6, 14, 11, 10, 12, 9, 12, 11, 8	$\bar{x}_A = 6.9, \bar{x}_B = 9.8$ $\bar{x}_B - \bar{x}_A = 2.9$
Week 14	6, 8, 7, 7, 4, 4, 7, 11, 8, 7, 7, 6, 12	9, 9, 6, 8, 12, 12, 11, 9, 6, 14, 11, 10, 12, 9, 12, 11, 8	$\bar{x}_A = 7.2, \bar{x}_B = 9.9$ $\bar{x}_B - \bar{x}_A = 2.7$

Step 4: Calculate the test statistic for all unused arrangements

If the null hypothesis is true and the intervention makes no difference to our observations, then dividing the observations at any point (including week 13) and comparing before and after means will just give random differences that are due to the intrinsic variation in our observations. But if the null hypothesis is not true and our intervention improves mobility, then subtracting the before mean from the after mean should give a larger difference when we divide at week 13 than if we divide at any other point.

This is the key to the randomization test. Table 2.5 gives the data with baseline and intervention means for the experiment, where week 13 was the intervention point. Also shown are the means for divisions at weeks 12 and 14, which would be part of the reference set.

To complete the reference set, we list the difference between before and after means with the division point at each of the possible intervention points from which we chose 13 at random, namely, points 6, 7, 8, 9 … up to 26. So for point 6 we need the difference between the mean of the last 25 observations and the first 5 observations, for point 7 we need the difference between the means of the last 24 and the first 6, and so on up to the difference between the means of the last 5 and the first 25. This list of differences between means is the reference set.

Step 5: Compare the actual statistic with those from the unused arrangements

How does the difference for point 13 compare with the others? Is it the biggest? Or one of the top two or three? If it's the biggest or near the top, then this may be evidence against the null hypothesis.

If it was the biggest, because we had 21 possible choices for our randomization (from point 6 to point 26), the probability of getting a result as good as this by chance is 1/21, which is less than 5%, so our result is significant at the 5% level. If our actual test statistic was only third from the top, then the probability of getting this by chance when the intervention has no effect (the null hypothesis) is 3/21 or 14.3%, and in this case we would not reject the null hypothesis that the intervention had no effect.

In this example, we used a one-tailed test because our alternative hypothesis was directional:

H_1: The intensive physiotherapy will improve mobility.

If our alternative was

H_1: The intensive physiotherapy will affect mobility, but we can't predict in which direction.

then we could use a two-tailed test and ignore the sign of the difference between the baseline and intervention means. As with parametric tests, two-tailed randomization tests are less powerful than one-tailed tests.

Phase designs: a single-case ABA design

Our example for the AB design is a case where withdrawal is not possible: If the intervention has any effect, it is likely to be long lasting. There are also cases where withdrawal may be possible but would not be ethically acceptable. However, here is an example where the intervention could be withdrawn.

Step 1: The example problem with the hypotheses

An educational psychologist suspects that a child with behavior problems may be made worse by some of the things he is eating. He and his mother agree to test the theory by removing from his diet for some days all foods containing sugar and food additives. They also agree that they will start the program on a day to be determined at random, and that on a later day, also determined at random, he will go back to his usual food and snacks until the end of the study. Our hypotheses are

H_0: The sugar- and additive-free diet will not affect behavior.
H_1: The sugar- and additive-free diet will improve behavior.

Four weeks (20 school days) are set aside for the study. The teacher will not be told which are the diet days, but at the end of each day will record a count of problem behavior that she observes. We decide that at least four observations are needed in each of the baseline and withdrawal

Table 2.6 Some of the Possible Days for Start and Withdrawal of Diet

No diet (Baseline)	Diet (Intervention)	No diet (Withdrawal)
1 2 3 4	5 6 7 8 9 10	11 12 13 14 15 16 17 18 19 20
1 2 3 4	5 6 7 8 9 10 11	12 13 14 15 16 17 18 19 20
1 2 3 4	5 6 7 8 9 10 11 12	13 14 15 16 17 18 19 20
1 2 3 4	5 6 7 8 9 10 11 12 13	14 15 16 17 18 19 20
1 2 3 4	5 6 7 8 9 10 11 12 13 14	15 16 17 18 19 20
1 2 3 4	5 6 7 8 9 10 11 12 13 14 15	16 17 18 19 20
1 2 3 4	5 6 7 8 9 10 11 12 13 14 15 16	17 18 19 20

phases where the child eats as normal, and at least six are needed for the diet days.

Step 2: Choose a random arrangement from those suitable

So the first diet day could be day 5, and it could be paired with returning to normal eating on day 17, 16, 15, 14, 13, 12, or 11. If day 5 as the first diet day is paired with day 17 as the first back-to-normal day, we have exactly four baseline and four withdrawal observations, and 12 diet days. The other pairs give more withdrawal days and fewer diet days, until day 5 and day 11 to start diet and withdrawal respectively give exactly 6 diet days. Table 2.6 shows the possible days for baseline, intervention, and withdrawal when day 5 is the first on the diet. Similarly, if day 6 is the first diet day, withdrawal can start on days 17, 16, 15, 14, 13, or 12. Day 7 can be paired with days 17, 16, 15, 14, or 13; day 8 can be paired with 17, 16, 15, or 14; day 9 with 17, 16, or 15,;day 10 with 17 or 16; and day 11 with day 17. If days 11 and 17 are used, we have 10 baseline and 4 withdrawal days, and 6 diet days.

We need to choose a pair of days for starting and withdrawing the diet. First list the possible pairs of days (there are 28), and then number the pairs from 1 to 28. There is an example of a systematic list of pairs of intervention and withdrawal points in Appendix 1. Now choose a random number between 1 and 28 to identify the pair to use. (Appendix 1 shows how to choose a random number in a range.) Suppose we choose at random the pair 7 (intervention) and 16 (withdrawal), so start the diet on day 7 and return to normal eating on day 16.

Step 3: Choose a test statistic

Our experiment gives us 11 baseline and withdrawal days, and 9 diet days. We are hoping the diet will reduce the problem behavior count, so a good choice of test statistic would be the mean score for nondiet days (all those in baseline and withdrawal) minus the mean score for diet days.

Table 2.7 Diet and No-Diet Means for Actual and Two Reference Set Divisions

Divide at	Baseline (A)	Intervention (B)	Withdrawal (A)	Means
Day 7 and 16 (actual)	12, 15, 14, 14, 9, 10	10, 16, 8, 11, 9, 5, 17, 8, 11	10, 10, 18, 17, 17	$\bar{x}_A = 13.3, \bar{x}_B = 10.6$ $\bar{x}_A - \bar{x}_B = 2.7$
Day 7 and 13	12, 15, 14, 14, 9, 10	10, 16, 8, 11, 9, 5	17, 8, 11, 10, 10, 18, 17, 17	$\bar{x}_A = 13.0, \bar{x}_B = 9.8$ $\bar{x}_A - \bar{x}_B = 3.2$
Day 10 and 16	12, 15, 14, 14, 9, 10, 10, 16, 8	11, 9, 5, 17, 8, 11	10, 10, 18, 17, 17	$\bar{x}_A = 12.9, \bar{x}_B = 10.2$ $\bar{x}_A - \bar{x}_B = 2.7$

Step 4: Calculate the test statistic for all unused arrangements

The null hypothesis is that the diet has no effect, and what if it is true? In that case, wherever we divide our observations into three blocks and calculate the mean of the beginning and end blocks to compare with the mean of the middle block (including the division we actually used), we shall be observing only random variation. If the diet does reduce the problem behavior count, then the difference between means from our experiment should be bigger than for any other division of the data. This is the key to the randomization test.

There are 27 other pairs of intervention and withdrawal points that we might have chosen during our random selection described above. For each of these, calculate the mean for the middle block and subtract it from the mean of the beginning and end blocks. These differences form the reference set. Table 2.7 shows the data with the test statistic for the experiment and two from the reference set.

Step 5: Compare the actual statistic with those from the unused arrangements

If the actual value we observed is the biggest, then either we chose at random the biggest of 28 with a probability of 1/28 or 3.6%, or else the diet did have an effect. If our result was only second biggest, the probability of getting that or better by chance would be 2/28 or 7%, so we would reject the null hypothesis only at the 5% level if our result is the biggest of the 28 possibilities.

Once again we used a one-tailed test, because our alternative hypothesis,

H_1: The sugar- and additive-free diet will improve behavior.

was directional.

If our alternative was

H_1: The sugar- and additive-free diet will affect behavior, but we can't predict in which direction.

then we could use a two-tailed test and ignore the sign of the difference between the baseline–withdrawal and intervention means. In this example, we would not be able to achieve a significant result with a two-tailed test.

Phase designs with multiple baselines

If we have an AB design with two or more cases, it is important to choose the intervention point at random for each case individually. This can be done by choosing a random number in the required range for the first case, then choosing another random number for the second case, and so on. Alternatively, we can list all possible sets of intervention points and choose a set at random.

For an ABA design with two or more cases, intervention and withdrawal points must be chosen at random individually for each case. The easiest way is to choose a pair of points for one case at a time and then repeat the process for the next case. These designs will be described fully in Chapter 4.

An example of order effects

Randomization tests can be devised to test for predicted orderings that are partial or complete. Here we consider an example of a predicted partial ordering.

Step 1: The example problem with the hypotheses

We are testing methods of helping students to cope with job interviews, and we have six volunteers to work with us. They will be randomly assigned to three methods of training, two volunteers to each method. The training will consist of

1. general advice about dress, punctuality, and self-presentation
2. the above, plus helping the student to think about the messages he or she wants to get across

or

3. both the above plus role playing with staff acting as an interview panel.

The university has advertised a job for which all these students are qualified, and we have requested that they all be interviewed, along with any other suitable applicants, and that the interview panel will tell us (and them) how they perform, arranging them in order as well as they can from best (6) to worst (1), allowing ties where they can't discriminate. We predict that the candidates who receive method 3 training will perform best, followed by those who receive method 2, and the worst performers will be those who receive method 1. So we are predicting a partial ordering, and our hypotheses are

H_0: The interview training will not affect interview performance.
H_1: The interview training methods 1, 2, and 3 will have increasing positive effects on interview performance.

If the data suggest that method 3 does improve performance, those volunteers who didn't get it will be offered it as thanks for their participation.

Step 2: Choose a random arrangement from those suitable
All we have to do here is assign the participants at random to the three methods (two to each). This is just the same as assigning the methods 1, 1, 2, 2, 3, and 3 in random order to the participants.

Step 3: Choose a test statistic
If method 3 results in the best performance (highest ranking), with method 2 next, and method 1 results in the worst performance (lowest ranking), the participants who received method 3 will have high performance rankings and those who received method 1 will get low rankings. If we multiply method number by performance ranking for each participant and add these products, the result will be a high value; whereas if performance rankings and method are not associated, the sum of products will be lower. This is the same idea as that used in calculating a correlation coefficient. So a suitable test statistic would be the sum of products of the method number and the interview ranking. (If we rank best to worst as 1 to 6 instead of 6 to 1, then we need to code the methods from 3 to 1 instead of 1 to 3, so that if H_1 is true, the sum of products will be large.)

Step 4: Calculate the test statistic for all unused arrangements
The null hypothesis is that the methods of training all have the same effect (if any) on performance, and if this is true then the training method is just an arbitrary label, and rearranging the labels will make no difference other than random variation to our test statistic. This is the key to the randomization test.

We have six labels, two each of 1, 2, and 3, so there are 6!/(2!2!2!) or 90 ways to arrange them. So we calculate the sum of products for the 89 unused arrangements to obtain the reference set. Table 2.8 shows the data with the test statistic for the experiment and also one from the reference set.

Step 5: Compare the actual statistic with those from the unused arrangements
If the test statistic from the actual experiment is in the top four (4.4% of 90) of the reference set, then we have a result that is significant at the 5% level: In this case, the evidence would suggest that the interview training methods 1, 2, and 3 have increasing positive effects on interview performance.

Table 2.8 Sum of Products for the Experiment on Order
Effects and One From the Reference Set

Student	Interviewers' order (y)	Training method (x)	Rearrangement (x)
1	4.5	2	2
2	1	1	3
3	2.5	2	1
4	6	3	1
5	4.5	3	3
6	2.5	1	2
		$\Sigma xy = 49$	$\Sigma xy = 39$

How randomization tests differ from more familiar tests

Our examples bring out several important aspects of randomization tests that distinguish them from conventional hypothesis tests such as t tests and ANOVAs. You may have noticed the first: We made no assumptions about the distribution of any observations—there's nothing comparable to assuming a set of measurements come from a Normal distribution, for instance. We also didn't assume our observations were a random sample from any population. In fact, our only assumption was that we assigned our experimental conditions at random to participants or observation occasions, or, to put it another way, we chose our arrangement of experimental conditions at random from those that were possible. In general, randomization tests make fewer assumptions than do more familiar parametric tests.

Another feature of randomization tests is that we can often stay close to our research question and find a test statistic that is a direct reflection of it. For the ESP experiment, this was the number of correctly identified test periods; for the factorial design and the phase designs, we used differences between condition means. Sometimes, as for the one-way design, we need a more complex summary of the data such as Fisher's F.

Probably the most important difference is the way in which we assess significance. When we calculate a t statistic, we assess statistical significance by comparing it with the t distribution. We can do this with a table, or if we use a package such as SPSS to get the t, it will also give the probability so we don't need to go to the table ourselves. But with our randomization designs, we compared the test statistic with the same statistic calculated from all the other arrangements that we did not use (the reference set). We have to calculate the values for the reference set ourselves each time we do a randomization test. Of course, we do use the macros for the calculations, but first we had to write them, and for new designs we would need new macros. We discuss this further in the next section.

Why randomization tests are not widely used

You might think that reducing the need for assumptions and often being able to choose an easily understandable test statistic would ensure that randomization tests were widely used. The difficulty in carrying out the procedures with an earlier generation of computers can perhaps explain why it has been slow to gain acceptance. But there are also two practical problems.

The first is that randomization tests are hard to generalize because we have to calculate the reference set ourselves. This is why statistical software such as SPSS doesn't usually provide for them. In this introductory text, we describe only nine designs (two with special cases and several that can be used with single cases or small groups), and for those we provide macros so that you can use SPSS or Excel for the analysis. We also suggest some ways in which you can expand your ability to deal with randomization tests once you master the basics.

The second problem is that we have to list the possible arrangements in order to calculate the test statistic for each one, and this can be a problem. Even if you know how many arrangements there are, making a list can be surprisingly difficult. Consider the 70 arrangements needed for the ESP experiment. Listing the 70 arrangements isn't just tedious but also very time consuming, and it's easy to make mistakes. You soon see this if you try making your own list. It's best to be systematic, and you could start like this:

```
VVVVNNNN
VVVNVNNN
VVNVVNNN
VNVVVNNN
NVVVVNNN
```

There are at least two sensible ways we could proceed from here: VVVNNVNN or NVVVNVNN. Listing a set of permutations is not simple even when you know how many there are. Some lists are short and easy (we only needed 20 for the factorial design), but some are much longer and correspondingly more difficult (210 for the one-way design). Even aided by fast computing, we need a strategy to deal with this problem, and in the next section we describe one.

If it's so difficult to list the permutations so that you can calculate the reference set, you may wonder how you are going to choose one at random to set up the experiment. Paradoxically, there is often an easy way to obtain one permutation at random without making a complete list, as we demonstrated in the section on hypothesis tests for ESP, one-way, and factorial examples. Where necessary, we include such details in our descriptions of our designs in Chapter 4.

Two ways to obtain the reference set

We have already mentioned that listing all possible arrangements in order to calculate the reference set can be difficult even if the list is not very long. This is not always so: For the single-case phase design, the list of possibilities for the randomization is very simple, just the intervention points from the end of the minimum baseline observations to the start of the minimum intervention observations. This is the easiest of all designs for which to calculate the reference set.

But for many designs making the list is difficult, and for some the total number of possible data arrangements is prohibitively large. If the number of test periods were to be doubled for the ESP experiment, the number of arrangements would be more than 600 million instead of 70. Even if we can't make a list, we can usually devise a simple way to choose one arrangement from it, as we did for several of the examples above. With eight test periods each of being viewed or not, we can use the coin toss method to choose one of the more than 600 million arrangements. Assign V for a head and N for a tail, and once you have eight of one of them, assign the last spaces to the other. Also, it is easy to arrange eight Vs and eight Ns in random order.

In cases where the number of arrangements is prohibitively large, it makes sense to take a random sample from all such arrangements and use this to obtain an approximation to the reference set. For the ESP experiment with eight each of V and N, we could easily obtain, say, 2000 arrangements by using 2000 random rearrangements of eight Vs and eight Ns, and this would give a good estimate of where the claimant's score stands compared with the reference set.

Even in cases where the number of arrangements is not very large, it may not be easy to list them, and then a good approximation to the reference set can be obtained by taking a large *random sample with replacement* from the possibilities. A random sample with replacement is one where, after an item is chosen, it is returned to the set of possibilities before the next item is chosen, so the set of possibilities is the same every time an item is chosen. A random sample *without replacement* is one where, once an item is chosen, it is removed from the set of possibilities so that it can't be chosen again. This means that every time an item is selected, the set of possibilities is reduced by one. If we are working with a large set of possibilities, it makes very little difference whether we sample with or without replacement, because removing one item from a large set doesn't change it much. In the next paragraph there is an explanation of how taking a random sample with replacement from the set of possible arrangements in our design works. It works just as well whether there are only a small number of arrangements (like the 70 in the ESP example), or a number much larger than our sample size of 1000 or 2000.

Think again about the ESP experiment with its 70 permutations. Imagine a sack containing a million (or even larger number of) copies of each of the 70 permutations. Now shake the sack and pull out a permutation at random. Count the number of correct answers. Put the permutation back in, shake again, and pull out the next. Count the number of correct answers. Repeat 1000, 2000, or however many times you decide is enough to give a good estimate of the proportion of permutations with at least as many correct as our claimant. Of course, we don't actually use the sack or physical copies, but the computer process we use is exactly equivalent. We just obtain a random arrangement of four Vs and four Ns 1000 or 2000 times using the computer. Similar methods can be devised for other randomization designs.

In order to have a consistent approach, in this book we obtain the reference set by using a random sample with replacement of 2000 arrangements from all those possible in the design, even in cases where it would be possible to make a complete list.

The number of arrangements needed for significance to be achievable

In our ESP example, there were 70 possible arrangements of the test periods. If we had only had three each of V and N, the number of possible arrangements would have been only 20. In this case, if our claimant got them all correct we would still have had a result that was just significant at 5% (1/20). However, if she got a less than perfect score even with four each of V and N, we couldn't reject the null hypothesis at the 5% level. We may want to design any experiment we do so that even if the effect we are looking for is not perfectly displayed, we would still have the possibility of getting a significant result. This shows that we need to take care when planning a design that we give ourselves sufficient opportunity to achieve significance. Even if the effect we are looking for is large and perfectly displayed by our experiment, we will still need at least 20 possibilities for the randomization. We consider this requirement in more detail for each design in Chapter 4, and more generally in Chapter 7, "Size and Power."

Exercises

1. Why is it difficult to include randomization tests in statistical software such as SPSS or Excel?
2. Why were randomization tests not developed much until fast computing was easily available?
3. In how many ways can the letters ABCD be arranged? List the arrangements.
4. In how many ways can the letters AABB be arranged? List the arrangements.
5. An AB design is required with at least four observations in each phase. The experimenter wants to be able to use a randomization test for the hypothesis that the intervention increases the scores. What would be the minimum number of observations that would allow the possibility of a result significant at the 5% level?
6. Why is the method of randomization part of the design?
7. Suggest two different methods of assigning at random the conditions for a 2*2 factorial design to 16 observation occasions with equal numbers in each condition.
8. Why is it important to assign the intervention point at random for each participant in a multiple baseline AB design?
9. What are the two ways to find out where our actual test statistic falls in the reference set?

chapter three

Obtaining the data
Choosing the design

Introduction

In this chapter we consider how to go about choosing a design for the problem we want to investigate. There are advantages and disadvantages to any design, and whatever we are investigating, we want to find a design that will address the question as directly as possible and that will have few disadvantages. We have to consider any factors that limit our choice of design, and if several types of design could be suitable, we need to be sure we know the advantages and disadvantages of each. In this introductory section, we briefly describe the classes of designs. Later sections will give the conditions in which each design may be used.

We are assuming in this book that the first limitation on our choice of design is that we don't have large numbers of participants, so we are unable to use the well-known formats and huge knowledge base available for large-sample designs. This limitation is implicit in the whole chapter, and indeed throughout the book, but in this introduction we look at some other possible limitations that may determine which designs are available to us.

Although we have said that having only one or a small group of participants is a limitation on our choice of design, we should point out that sometimes there is particular value in finding out what happens to a few individual cases. Large-sample designs tell us about average effects, and there will always be variation in individual response. So we can take a positive view of single-case and small-*n* designs: They teach us about individuals and have an important place in research in the human sciences, as we explained in Chapter 1.

Many years of development have given us large-sample designs that ensure our results will not be tainted by observer bias or group selection bias, or be swamped in uncontrolled random variation. In the less well-trodden ways of small-*n* and single-case designs, we need to make sure we have attended to these issues. Because of this, we give a brief account of *internal* and *external validity* here in the introduction, but we also mention validity when describing those particular designs for which validity may be problematic. We revisit this topic in Chapter 6.

Types of experimental design

We consider three classes of experimental design, as we explained in Chapter 2. The first class comprises those designs that are analogs of ANOVA. These are the most powerful designs and will be the best choice if we can find one that is suitable. Unfortunately, as the next section explains, there are plenty of situations where none of them is appropriate.

Phase designs are our next group, and as we shall see, one of them may be the design of last resort. It is often hard to ensure internal validity, as we explain in the case of the AB design below. These designs usually also have low power (in other words, they may have a high probability of missing an effect that is real), an issue we discuss in Chapter 7. Nevertheless, one of these designs could be the way to move an investigation forward, and in that case it is important to make sure the design is as good as we can make it.

We also consider order effects, though designs to examine these can sometimes be criticized as not being proper randomization designs. We show the kind of problem to which they are applied in this chapter, and we discuss their place in the scheme of randomization designs in Chapter 6.

Examples that can be used with either a small group or a single case are available for each of our classes of randomization designs: analogs of ANOVA, phase designs, and order effects. We now look at some features that may restrict our choice of design before concluding this introduction with a discussion of validity.

Limits to our choice of design

Our choice of design may often be limited by what kind of randomization is possible with the conditions we want to compare. Can the conditions we want to compare be randomly assigned to participants (if we have a small group) or to observation occasions (if we have a single case)? An example where the conditions could be randomly assigned would be the three methods of pain control in the single-case one-way design in Chapter 2. It does not matter if the conditions precede or follow one of the other methods of pain control because the pain control methods can be effective only while they are being used. They could therefore be assigned at random to the available observation periods for a single case, or if we had a group of eligible participants, the methods could be randomly assigned to them. A design analogous to ANOVA can usually be used if this kind of random assignment is possible.

There are some conditions or treatments that cannot be randomly assigned to observation periods. An example is an intervention such as surgery or a training course that has a long-lasting or permanent effect. If this is the subject of investigation, then the only option may be a before-and-after study, a phase design.

For some conditions or treatments, we may be in some doubt about whether random assignment to observation occasions is possible or appropriate. Our example for a phase design with a reversal phase in Chapter 2 is such a case. Here the conditions were normal food or a diet free from sugar and additives, and the observation occasions were school days. It would be possible to randomly assign the diet or normal food to each observation day, but there are two reasons why we may prefer not to do that if it can be avoided. First, it may be easier for our participant to stick to the diet for a block of consecutive days than for days assigned at random among normal food days. We do need his full compliance, so we should avoid making it harder than necessary for him. But also, it is possible that there is a short carry over effect from either a diet day or a normal food day into the next day. If there is, random assignment would allow this effect to obscure our results. The phase design we adopted would minimize any damage done to our results by a short carry over effect. In fact, if we believed such a thing might prejudice our results, we could decide, as part of the design, that the data from the first diet day and the first withdrawal day would be ignored.

As these examples illustrate, the first thing we have to consider when choosing a design is what limitations are imposed on the way we use randomization by the conditions or treatments we want to investigate. Other limitations may be imposed by our participants' ability or willingness to attend observation sessions, or record measurements or observations themselves. Some designs, especially phase designs, may require an unacceptably long series of observations. Cost can also impose limits on the number or type of observations that are possible.

Ethical considerations can also limit our choice of design, and the same constraints apply to small-n and single-case designs as to large-sample ones. Of particular relevance to us is the likelihood of being unable to use a phase design with reversal because if the participant becomes accustomed to, or benefits from, the intervention, then withdrawing it may be impossible.

Internal and external validity

When we set up an experiment to compare the effects of two or more conditions or treatments, we want to be able to say that any observed difference must be due to the different conditions or treatments, and cannot be explained by such things as observer bias or preexisting differences among participants. This is the requirement that we attend to *internal validity*, and many threats to it have been uncovered over the years, including the placebo effect, unconscious or conscious observer bias, and unconsidered differences among participants. Even though randomization tests require fewer assumptions than parametric tests, careful consideration of possible threats to internal validity is just as important a part of choosing a design and setting up an experiment as it is for a large-sample experiment.

External validity refers to the general application of any result found: Most results are of little interest unless they can be applied to a wider population than those taking part in the experiment. External validity may be claimed if those taking part were a random sample from the population to which we want to generalize the results. In practice, when people are the subjects of experiments, as well as in many other situations, random sampling is an unrealistic ideal, and external validity is achieved by repeating the experiment in other contexts. This applies equally to large-sample experiments and the small-*n* and single-case experiments that are the subject of this book.

In the interests of internal validity, we often use "blinding" of participants or assessors to the condition being applied. Here is how it is used in a large randomized controlled trial, which has become the gold standard for comparing the efficacy of treatments. Eligible participants are randomly assigned to one of the treatments or else to the control group (which may receive an already established treatment). Normally, neither the participants nor their assessors know to which group they have been assigned, because many subtle effects have been found that are mediated by either the experimenters' or participants' beliefs about the treatments. So only the administrator, who never sees the participants, holds the key to who received which treatment. Sometimes considerable efforts must be made to make pills look alike or otherwise blind participants and experimenters to the treatment being received. This type of design generally removes any threat to internal validity.

With small groups or single cases, we usually have to modify the large-sample approach to achieving internal validity. In several of the descriptions below, we draw attention to how internal validity may be compromised and the kind of efforts we can make to improve it.

Choosing the randomization method

Before we consider example designs, there is one more general point to emphasize: When we do the randomization to obtain the reference set, we must use the same method as for setting up the experiment. The ESP example from Chapter 2 will show what we mean. We decided to assign four each of conditions V and N randomly to the eight test periods. The randomization can easily be achieved by arranging four Vs and four Ns in random order as shown in Appendix 1. We could also toss a coin as shown in Chapter 2.

We chose to have equal numbers in the two conditions, but you may have wondered whether an equally good method would be to perform the coin toss for every test period and use the number of Vs and Ns thus obtained. This might make our ESP claimant's task harder, because she will no longer know that there are four of each, so perhaps this variant of the design would be an improvement. Remember that to set up the randomization test, we must calculate the test statistic for all the unused random assignments, the rest of the reference set. What would they be, and how many are there if we do it this way? Each of the eight test periods can be one of two conditions, so the first two have 2*2 possible assignments (VV, VN, NV, and NN). The first three have 2*2*2 possible assignments (VVV, VVN, VNV, NVV, VNN, NVN, NNV, and NNN). The eight test periods have $2^8 = 256$ possible assignments. Two of these would be all V or all N, so we may wish to reject them, leaving 254 possible assignments. We can obtain the reference set by listing them and counting the number correct for each assignment (compared with the one actually used), or else we can sample with replacement as described in Chapter 2. If we use the sampling method, generating each assignment by the computer equivalent of coin tossing, we need to make sure we reject the cases with all Vs or all Ns from the reference set if we exclude them from the design. This example illustrates the importance of deciding just how the randomization is to be done when choosing the design, and also how the reference set must be obtained using the same method of randomization.

In most circumstances, we shall want to collect equal or nearly equal numbers of observations in each condition, because the more nearly equal the numbers, the more powerful the test will be. However, for several designs the numbers do not *need* to be equal and may depend on constraints beyond our control. If one of the conditions is expensive or difficult to arrange, there may be a limit to the number of observations we can obtain for it, but it may be worth collecting a few more for the other conditions. In our example on pain control in Chapter 2, for instance, if the acupuncturist has a very full appointment book, we may be able to arrange only a small number of appointments within the time scale of the experiment. We now consider the uses, advantages, and disadvantages of the individual designs, grouped into their classes.

Designs analogous to ANOVA

If the treatments or conditions under investigation are suitable for random assignment to participants or observation occasions, then a design analogous to one of those used with ANOVA for large-*n* designs will give the best opportunity to demonstrate any effect. This flexible class of designs enables us to compare two or more treatments or conditions. We can also incorporate repeated measures as well as consider two factors in a single experiment. This is as far as we go in this book, but randomization designs analogous to more complex ANOVAs could be devised using the five steps described in Chapter 2.

A single-case one-way design

This design is appropriate when the following conditions apply:

1. We have only one participant.
2. There are several available observation occasions that are all equivalent.
3. We have two or more conditions to compare.
4. It is possible to assign conditions to observation occasions at random.

Condition 2 would not be satisfied if, for instance, we are obliged to use both mornings and afternoons to obtain enough observation occasions, but we suspect that our participant will respond differently in the morning and afternoon. Likewise, it would not apply if we have to use two observers, and we suspect there may be slight differences in the way they make their assessments. If condition 2 does not apply, we need to consider a single-case randomized blocks design.

Condition 4 would not be satisfied if any of the conditions has a lasting or permanent effect, so that the next observation occasion would be affected by a condition applied previously. So this design might enable us to compare painkilling drugs, but not different surgical interventions. For investigating a long-lasting or permanent intervention, a phase design should be considered.

If there are only two conditions to compare, we can use a special case of this design that makes a one-tailed test possible. The macro is the same as the one for a small-*n* one-way design with two conditions and is described in Chapter 4.

As always with a single-case design, external validity will be achieved only after similar results are found with other participants in other contexts.

A small-n one-way design

This design is appropriate when the following conditions apply:

1. We have at least two participants.
2. Each participant will be measured once only.
3. We have two or more conditions to compare.
4. It is possible to assign conditions to participants at random.

Condition 2 will not apply if our investigation requires a series of two or more measurements on each participant, perhaps to record a process. In this case, a small-*n* repeated measures design should be considered. However, condition 2 could apply if the single measurement recorded for each participant is actually an average from several raters or observers.

Condition 4 of course implies that all participants are suitable and willing to be assigned to any of the conditions. Because each participant is observed only once, this time we may be less concerned if any of the conditions has a long-lasting effect.

If there are only two conditions to compare, we can use a special case of this design that makes a one-tailed test possible. This special case is described in Chapter 4 as a small-*n* one-way design with two conditions.

A single-case randomized blocks design

This design is appropriate when the following conditions apply:

1. We have only one participant.
2. The available observation occasions fall into two or more groups (days, for instance).
3. We have two or more conditions to compare.
4. It is possible to assign conditions to observation occasions at random.

We use a randomized blocks design if we are collecting data at several times, perhaps on different days, to reduce the chance of any treatment effect being obscured by variation among observation occasions. So, in case our participant has good and bad days, we can apply each treatment in random order within each day (block), so differences among treatments will be found within each block and then averaged over blocks. This is just the same idea that motivates randomized block designs for use with ANOVA.

As in the single-case one-way design, condition 4 will not apply if any of the conditions has a long-lasting or permanent effect.

If there are only two conditions to compare, we can use a special case of this design that makes a one-tailed test possible. This special case is described in Chapter 4 as a single-case randomized blocks design with two conditions.

As always with a single-case design, external validity will be achieved only after similar results are found with other participants in other contexts.

A small-n repeated measures design

This design is appropriate when the following conditions apply:

1. We have at least two participants.
2. We have two or more conditions to compare.

3. Each participant will receive each of the conditions.
4. It is possible to assign conditions in random order to each participant.

Because human participants are usually very variable, we may improve our ability to detect differences among the conditions by finding the differences within each participant and averaging the results. In this way, each participant acts as their own control. The same idea is used in repeated measures designs for large groups.

Condition 4 will not apply if any of the conditions has a long-lasting effect, just as in the single-case one-way and randomized blocks designs. This is again because a long-lasting effect would influence the next observation.

If there are only two conditions to compare, we can use a special case of this design that makes a one-tailed test possible. The macro is the same as the one used for the single-case randomized blocks design with two conditions, described in Chapter 4.

A small-n repeated measures design with replicates

This design is appropriate when the following conditions apply:

1. We have at least two participants.
2. We have two conditions to compare.
3. Each participant will receive each of the conditions on at least two occasions.
4. It is possible to assign conditions in random order to each participant.

As in the previous design, here each participant acts as his or her own control. As long as we have only two conditions to compare, we can use this design to improve our chance of finding a significant effect. Our macro assumes that we have equal numbers of observations in each condition and the same number of observations for each participant. The conditions will be assigned in random order to each participant.

Condition 4 will not apply if any of the conditions has a long-lasting effect, just as in the single-case one-way and randomized blocks designs. This is again because a long-lasting effect would influence the next observation.

It is possible to use the macro for this design for a randomized blocks design with replicates, and this use is outlined in Chapter 4.

A two-way factorial single-case design

Factorial designs allow us to investigate two or more variables in a single experiment. Here we consider only the two-way factorial, which means we consider two variables. An example would be an experiment to investigate the effectiveness of different types of painkilling drug and also different relaxation methods (using music or exercise, perhaps). The two-way design described here allows just two levels for each variable (two drugs and two relaxation methods in the example just outlined).

This two-way factorial design is appropriate when the following conditions apply:

1. We have a single participant.
2. A series of observation occasions is available.
3. We have two factors to investigate (for instance, drug type and relaxation method).
4. There are two levels of each factor (for instance, drugs A and B, and relaxation methods X and Y).
5. It is possible to assign conditions in random order to observation occasions.

Notice that there are four conditions here (AX, BX, AY, and BY). We shall need equal numbers of observations for the four conditions, so will use 4, 8, 12, or some other multiple of four observation occasions. Condition 5 will not apply if any of the treatments has a long-lasting or permanent effect.

By observing a single participant, we remove the variability among participants, but as always with a single-case design, external validity will accumulate only as the experiment is repeated with different people in different situations.

A two-way factorial small-n design

This design is appropriate when the following conditions apply:

1. We have a multiple of four participants.
2. We have two factors to investigate (for instance, drug type and relaxation method).
3. There are two levels of each factor (for instance, drugs A and B, and relaxation methods X and Y).
4. It is possible to assign conditions at random to participants.

Each participant will receive one of the four conditions (AX, AY, BX, or BY). Because each is measured only once, condition 4 may still apply even if a condition has a long-lasting effect. Of course, all participants must be suitable and willing to receive any of the conditions.

Phase designs

Phase designs have their own particular problems with internal validity, because inevitably time passes during the study, and many things change with time. A phase design with *reversal* may help with this problem:

It is one where, after we have sufficient measurements in the intervention phase, we withdraw the intervention and continue taking measurements for the *withdrawal phase*. This is known as an ABA design. Of course, this is not always possible: There may be ethical reasons why we cannot withdraw a drug or therapy once offered, especially if the participant seems to be benefiting. Also our intervention may be irreversible, as would be the case if it took the form of surgery or a training session. However, evidence that any observed effect was due to the intervention may be strengthened if a reversal phase is possible.

Another problem with phase designs is that successive observations may be correlated, especially if the time between observations is short. Imagine recording blood pressure daily. Now imagine recording it every 10 minutes. If you record every 10 minutes, successive measurements are likely to be similar. If you record it daily, then successive measurements are less likely to be similar. If successive observations are similar, the effect is called *serial correlation*, and we show how to check for this in Appendix 1. Every effort should be made to ensure that the serial correlation is low, and this will mean that sufficient time must be allowed between observations. Another opportunity for reducing serial correlation concerns the way in which observations are made: When the same individual makes repeated measurements, there may be an increased chance of serial correlation. This might be avoided by assigning different raters at random to observation periods, but then unless interrater reliability is high we might introduce unnecessary extra variability into the data.

Phase designs qualify as randomization designs only if intervention and withdrawal points are chosen at random from those available. This is not the traditional way to implement a phase design, but doing the randomization not only allows us to use a randomization test but also removes a threat to internal validity. We expand on this point, and provide some evidence that even quite experienced researchers can be misled, in Chapter 6.

The single-case AB design

This design is appropriate when the following conditions apply:

1. We have a single participant.
2. We want to test the effectiveness of an intervention.
3. A series of observations is possible both before and after the intervention.
4. It is possible to choose the intervention point at random.

Conditions 3 and 4 will not apply if the participant urgently needs the intervention and cannot wait for a randomly assigned time to receive it.

This is the simplest of the phase designs, and the choice to use this design is often determined by the irreversible or long-lasting nature of the intervention being investigated: In fact, it may be the design of last resort. Nevertheless, it may move our investigation forward, and we need to make sure we do it as well as possible. Randomizing the intervention point is the first step.

The single-case ABA design

This design is appropriate when the following conditions apply:

1. We have a single participant.
2. We want to test the effectiveness of an intervention.
3. After sufficient observations are obtained, it will be possible to withdraw the intervention.
4. A series of observations is possible before the intervention, while the intervention continues, and after it is withdrawn.
5. It is possible to choose the intervention and withdrawal points at random.

Conditions 4 and 5 will not apply if the participant urgently needs the intervention, just as in the AB design. Condition 3 will not apply if the intervention is irreversible, such as surgery or training. It will also not apply if there are ethical objections to withdrawal.

If withdrawal is possible, the extra randomization will reduce the total number of observations needed. This effect can be seen in the examples used in Chapter 2 but will be shown in more detail in Chapter 4, where we implement the designs.

In addition to reducing the number of observations needed, the addition of a withdrawal phase may increase our confidence in the effectiveness of the intervention if the effect disappears when the intervention is withdrawn. The additional persuasive power of the withdrawal phase may be a strong reason to use this design if it is possible.

If a reversal phase is possible, then it may be useful to add a further intervention phase, giving us an ABAB design, and even more phases can be added. We can also have phase designs with two different interventions with a withdrawal phase in between, giving an ABAC design. You can think of more variants yourself, but multiple phases are more likely to lead to ethical problems, and implementation and analysis may also be more difficult. We discuss some of these possibilities further in Chapter 8.

The multiple baseline AB design

This design is appropriate when the following conditions apply:

1. We have at least two participants (a variant for one participant is given below).
2. We want to test the effectiveness of an intervention.
3. For each participant, a series of observations is possible both before and after the intervention.
4. It is possible to choose the intervention point at random for each participant.

Using the AB design with two or more participants will substantially reduce the number of observations needed on each participant, which may be a considerable advantage. However, it is important that the intervention point is chosen at random individually for each participant. Condition 4 will not apply if the intervention has to start at the same time for all participants.

If we find a significant effect, we shall be able to say only that the intervention produced a significant effect for at least one of the participants. We shall have to rely on visual inspection to suggest which ones showed the effect.

Conditions 3 and 4 will not apply if any participant needs the intervention urgently, just as in the single-case AB design.

This design may also be used with a single participant if we want to test the effectiveness of several interventions during a single series of observation occasions. An example of this use is given in Chapter 4.

The multiple baseline ABA design

This design is appropriate when the following conditions apply:

1. We have at least two participants (but see the note at the end for one participant).
2. We want to test the effectiveness of an intervention.
3. After sufficient observations are obtained, it will be possible to withdraw the intervention.
4. For each participant, a series of observations is possible before the intervention, while the intervention continues, and after it is withdrawn.
5. It is possible to choose the intervention and withdrawal points at random.

Using the ABA design with two or more participants will substantially reduce the number of observations needed on each participant, which may be an advantage. However, it is important that the intervention and withdrawal points are chosen at random individually for each participant. Condition 5 will not apply if intervention and withdrawal have to start at the same time for all participants.

If we find a significant effect, we shall only be able to say that the intervention produced a significant effect for at least one of the participants. We shall have to rely on visual inspection to suggest which.

Condition 3 will not apply if the intervention is irreversible or if there are ethical problems with withdrawal. Conditions 4 and 5 will not apply if any participant needs the intervention urgently.

As with the multiple baseline AB design, this design may be used with a single participant if we can take more than one type of measurement on each observation occasion, if each measurement has an associated intervention to be tested, and if the interventions can be made at individually chosen random points.

Advantages of phase designs

Phase designs allow us to investigate treatments or therapies with which we hope to help people who have rare or very individual disorders or disabilities. We may never have even a small group of people with a particular set of problems, much less the numbers needed for a conventional clinical trial. But still, we want to make as good and as objective an assessment as possible of any proposed intervention. A phase design may be the only option, and if so, using randomization of the intervention point gives the best hope of avoiding bias and demonstrating effectiveness using statistical significance.

Disadvantages of phase designs

Double-blind randomized controlled trials were developed to avoid the pitfalls that bedevil attempts to assess the effectiveness of treatments, including observer bias and the placebo effect. Phase designs usually are open to some of these problems. If the intervention is a drug, then the placebo effect may be countered if the participant can be given a dated strip of pills that all look alike, so the participant doesn't know when the intervention starts. Even then, the occurrence of side effects from the drug may let the participant know when the intervention starts. For other kinds of intervention such as training or surgery, where the participant inevitably knows when it occurs, we may not be able to distinguish an effect from the passing effect of optimism or novelty. Considering this possibility may influence our choice of the minimum acceptable number of observations in the intervention phase, and it might help if we exclude from the analysis the first few observations immediately after the intervention. We may be able to reduce opportunities for observer bias by having someone unaware of when the intervention occurs taking the measurements.

The need for a long series of observations may be a problem, either because it is tedious for the participant or because the measurement may be affected by boredom or practice. If the necessity of avoiding highly correlated neighboring observations, or other constraints of the study, means that observations are quite widely spaced (e.g., perhaps once a week), then we have to consider whether the mere passage of time, over more than half a year perhaps, may bring about changes that will obscure the effect of our intervention.

Finally, if we want to use statistical tests on these designs, we have to be aware that they can be quite insensitive to small effects. In other words, we might not find enough evidence to support effects that are really there. We discuss this issue in Chapter 7 on size and power.

A design to investigate order effects

This design is appropriate when the following conditions apply:

1. We have a single participant and several observation occasions, or else several participants.
2. We want to test whether two variables are correlated.
3. Both variables are at least ordered.
4. It is possible to assign values of one of the variables at random to participants or observation occasions.

Condition 3 will not apply if one of the variables is something like POLITICAL AFFILIATION, with categories such as LABOUR, CONSERVATIVE, GREEN, LIBERAL, and OTHER, because these categories are not ordered. A variable such as FREQUENCY, with categories DAILY, WEEKLY, MONTHLY, and LESS THAN ONCE A MONTH, is ordered and so could be used here. Of course, any measurement is ordered and can also be used.

Condition 4 applies to something like number of training sessions, which could be randomly assigned to participants, but not to something like age, which is an unalterable property of a participant and so cannot be assigned at random.

Here is the kind of problem addressed by this design: One variable can be assigned at random (number of training sessions perhaps), and the other variable, which may be correlated, will be measured on each participant (performance score on a task, for instance). Then, we can test whether or not the two variables are correlated or not.

It is possible to use this design even if there are ties in the ordering of one of the variables. For instance, instead of using the number of training hours, suppose we have just three training methods that are ordered by intensity. Assuming we have more than three participants, there will inevitably be ties in the ordering of the training method variable. If the methods can be randomly assigned to a small group of participants, then we can still investigate the possible association of training method with performance on a task. Our example in Chapter 2 was of this type. It is also possible to have ties on a variable because participants get equal scores or ratings on whatever is being observed.

Exercises

1. Why is it difficult to ensure internal validity for phase designs?
2. If we use a single-case or small-*n* design with no random sampling, how can external validity be achieved?
3. If we want to assess the effectiveness of a surgical intervention using a single participant, which designs may be suitable?
4. We need a design to compare four conditions. We shall be able to make only four observations per day. Why might we consider a randomized block rather than a one-way design?
5. If we have a small group of suitable participants who are willing to be randomly assigned to one of two conditions, either a surgical intervention or a period of observation with no treatment, which designs should we consider? Suggest a way in which we might encourage patients to participate, and also a way to improve internal validity.
6. If we are investigating the effectiveness of a possible treatment for a single participant, what considerations will influence our choice of design?
7. Are there conditions in which a multiple baseline phase design would be preferable to a small-*n* one-way or repeated measures design?

chapter four

Obtaining the data
Implementing the design

Introduction

If the last chapter enabled you to choose a design that suits your investigation, this one will show you exactly how to implement it. This includes details of how to carry out the randomizations. You may need to refer to Appendix 1 if you are not confident with the random number facilities in your chosen analysis package, but we will draw attention to this when necessary. Chapter 5 shows how to analyze the designs using our macros in either SPSS or Excel and gives the results for the examples used here.

It is important that the data are set out correctly for the macros, and we show how to do this using example data. The layout of the datasets is the same for SPSS and Excel, except that in the Excel worksheet the first row is devoted to variable names. SPSS holds the names above the datasheet. It is important that you use the same variable names as in the examples when you use the macros with your own data. You can download the example datasets used in this chapter from the book Web site (http://www.researchmethodsarena.com/9780415886932). You may want to use these as templates for your own data: You can easily edit them, removing the example data and replacing it with your own. Just open the required example data file in your chosen package, delete the data but leave the variable names unchanged, and enter your own data. (For four of the Excel macros, it is also necessary to edit the range of names used by the macro. There are instructions for this in Appendix 3.)

In our first example, we show the SPSS and Excel datasheets as well as a data table, so that you can see exactly how they correspond. For later examples we give only the data table. Also in the first example, we show how to calculate the number of possible arrangements using a calculator, but in subsequent examples we don't show the calculator steps. We give more detail on performing the randomization for the first example than for later ones. Even if you are interested in using one of the other designs, we urge you to read the first example carefully, so that you see all these details before using one of the briefer accounts to guide your own work.

We give some explanation of our choice of test statistics. You can just assume these choices are sensible (you never have to calculate them yourself because the macros will do it for you), or you can try to follow our reasons for the choice. Sometimes more than one sensible choice would be possible, and then we prefer one that is convenient for the macro to calculate. For some of the designs analogous to ANOVA, you will understand the choice of test statistic better if you have a fairly good knowledge of ANOVA, but you can use the macros without this if you trust our choice.

We explain how the reference set is obtained by the macro, and you may notice that the way randomizations are done to get the reference set always matches the randomization used for the design. Understanding this will enhance your grasp of randomization tests, but you don't need to be able to obtain the reference set for yourself. However, if later on you want to try editing our macros or writing new ones for other designs, you will certainly want to know what we did.

We show how to calculate the number of possible arrangements for each design so that you can check whether you have enough for a significant result to be possible. However, if you are not confident with these calculations, here is another way to find out. When you think your design is satisfactory, make up some pseudo-data for it that is obviously incompatible with the null hypothesis, for example put in scores where there is no overlap between different conditions. Then run the appropriate macro with the pseudo-data and see if you obtain a significant result. If you don't get a significant result with pseudo-data that is obviously incompatible with the null hypothesis, then however the experiment turns out, your real data will not give a significant result, and you should look at ways to increase your number of observations or participants.

Designs analogous to ANOVA

As explained in Chapter 3, these designs may be used only if the treatments or conditions to be investigated can be randomly assigned to participants or observation occasions.

We provide extra macros for the special case when there are only two conditions to compare in a one-way design (single-case or small-*n*): a small-*n* randomized blocks design or a single-case repeated-measures design, so that a directional alternative may be used, as described in the next paragraph.

If there are only two conditions, it may be possible to have a directional alternative hypothesis, as in our factorial example where we had two levels for factor 1, carer present or absent. The null hypothesis is that the presence of the carer makes no difference, but the alternative is that disruptive behavior is *reduced* when the carer is present. For the designs with only two conditions, the test statistic is the condition 2 mean minus the condition 1 mean. To use the one-tailed probability, you must code the conditions so that condition 2 is predicted to give the higher mean.

We give examples for the single-case and small-*n* one-way designs for the general case, but for the special case of just two conditions we give only a small-*n* example. The macro and the analysis are the same for a single case or a small group in both the general case and the special case. The macro for the special case of two conditions is also used for investigating the simple effects in a 2*2 factorial design.

There is also a single macro for the single-case randomized blocks and small-*n* repeated-measures designs, but we give an example of its use for each. As for the one-way design, there is also an extra macro for the special case with only two conditions, and we give just one example for that.

The factorial design and its macro can be used with a single case or small group, and we give an example of each.

If there are three or more conditions, a directional alternative is not possible. All we can ask is whether the scores are different across conditions or not. Where we have provided an extra macro for the case of just two conditions (the one-way, small-*n* repeated-measures and single-case randomized blocks designs), the general macro can be used with only two conditions, but if we want to use a directional alternative, then we have to use the macro for the special case of just two conditions.

For the calculations of the number of possible arrangements, there is an extra step for designs with more than two conditions. In these cases, the test statistic has to treat all the conditions in the same way (we use the residual sum of squares like in ANOVA). This means that, when we calculate the number of possible arrangements, we have to allow for the fact that rearranging condition labels among equal-sized groups would not affect the test statistic, because all conditions are treated in the same way. This is a subtle point, and if you are not confident with calculating the number of possible arrangements, then take the easy way out suggested at the end of the introduction to this chapter.

A single-case one-way design

Our example

We want to encourage a patient with Alzheimer's disease to join in activities, and we want to find out if having music during the activity will help. We have three methods to test: loud music (L), soft music (S), and quiet (Q). The patient attends a day center three times a week, and we can use three weeks, or nine sessions, for the study. Three sessions will be assigned at random to each method. Five activities are arranged for each session, and our participant will be given a score for the number of activities he joins in.

Decisions to make

The decisions to make before this design can be implemented are as follows:

1. How many treatments or conditions are to be included in the experiment, including the control if there is one (our example has three)
2. How many observation occasions are available (our example has nine)
3. How many observation occasions will be allocated to each treatment (three, three, and three in our example)

We do not need equal numbers of measurements on the treatments, but equal or nearly equal numbers will give the best chance of a significant result.

We should check that all the observation occasions are similar: If they are not, perhaps a single-case randomized blocks design would be more suitable. In our example, we would consider this if different carers organize the activities on different days of the week. But in our example, this is unnecessary as the organizer is always the same on the days our participant attends.

Calculating the number of possible arrangements

We need to check that the number of possible arrangements of treatments over the observation occasions makes a significant result a possibility: Twenty arrangements would be an absolute minimum for significance at the 5% level to be possible. Chapter 2 includes a section on calculating the number of arrangements, but here are the details of the calculations for our example. We can do this check on any scientific calculator: Look for the factorial symbol $x!$, which may be above one of the keys so that you need to use the **Shift** key. We have 3 conditions (treatments) and will assign 3 of each to 9 observation occasions, giving $9!/(3!3!3!)$ possible arrangements. Enter **9** on the calculator, then $x!$ and find 362880 on the screen. To divide by 3!, press ÷ then **3** then $x!$, so we now have 60480. Divide by 3! again and get 10080. Finally, divide by 3! for the third time and get 1680, the number of possible arrangements of the 3 treatments (each given 3 times) over the 9 observation occasions.

This looks promising, but, as we mentioned at the end of the introduction to this section, we have to allow for the fact that rearranging the condition labels would not alter the test statistic. There are 3! or 6 ways to arrange the 3 letters L, S, and Q among themselves, so the number of arrangements giving distinct test statistics will be the 1680 we calculated in the previous paragraph divided by 6, or 280. This is plenty to allow the possibility of significance at the 5% level (1/280 is about 0.4%).

The same method can be applied whatever the numbers of occasions and conditions. We do have a large enough set of possible arrangements: We would achieve a result significant at the 5% level if our result is one of the top 14 (5% of 280).

Performing the randomization

There are usually several ways to do the randomization for a design. Listing the possible arrangements and choosing one at random is hardly ever the most convenient, even in a case where the list is not very long. The most convenient method in this example is to number the conditions 1, 2, and 3 and then get SPSS or Excel to arrange 1, 1, 1, 2, 2, 2, 3, 3, and 3 in random order (because we need three of each condition). Appendix 1, "Basic Skills for Randomization Tests," shows how to do this and other methods of randomization.

It may be worth emphasizing that for this design we decided in advance how many observation occasions are to be allocated to each condition, so a randomization method where this is selected randomly would be incorrect. An example of incorrect randomization would be choosing nine random numbers between 1 and 3 (for example, 3, 2, 3, 1, 2, 1, 3, 3, and 3). This result would then determine how many observation occasions each condition gets (two each of 1 and 2, and five 3s in this case). A one-way design using this latter method of randomization is possible, but we have not considered it here or provided a macro for it. So, in general, it is important to match the randomization procedure used for the experiment to the one used in the macro.

Now we apply the conditions in the random order we obtained to the 9 days. We coded quiet as 1, soft music as 2, and loud music as 3. Our random order for the conditions was 2, 1, 2, 1, 3, 1, 3, 3, and 2. So taking the 9 days in order, we use soft music for day 1, then quiet for day 2, then soft music and so on until finally soft music on day 9.

The datasheet

Our counts of the patient joining in activities on the successive days were 2, 1, 4, 3, 3, 2, 3, 4, and 3. The results must now be arranged in the SPSS datasheet or the Excel worksheet as shown in Table 4.1, with the condition 1 counts followed by condition 2 and so on, rather than in the order in which they were collected. The number in column 1, labeled "limits," is the number of observations. The example data shown here can be found on the book Web site as *onewaysinglecase.sav* (SPSS) or *oneway.xlsm* (Excel). Figure 4.1 shows the datasheet as it appears in SPSS (Figure 4.1a) and in Excel (Figure 4.1b). Remember to use the same variable names as shown here.

Table 4.1 Datasheet for One-Way Single-Case Design

Limits	Data	Condition
9	1	1
	3	1
	2	1
	2	2
	4	2
	3	2
	3	3
	3	3
	4	3

The test statistic

In this section, we give a brief explanation of our choice of test statistic. The macro will do all the calculations, so you can just accept that our choice is sensible. But if you want a better understanding of it, you need to know a bit about analysis of variance (ANOVA). Most statistics books cover this, for example Howell (2010) or Dugard et al. (2010).

Because we have three conditions to compare, we can't use a difference between two means as our test statistic. We need a summary of our data that shows up the differences among condition means, and Fisher's F

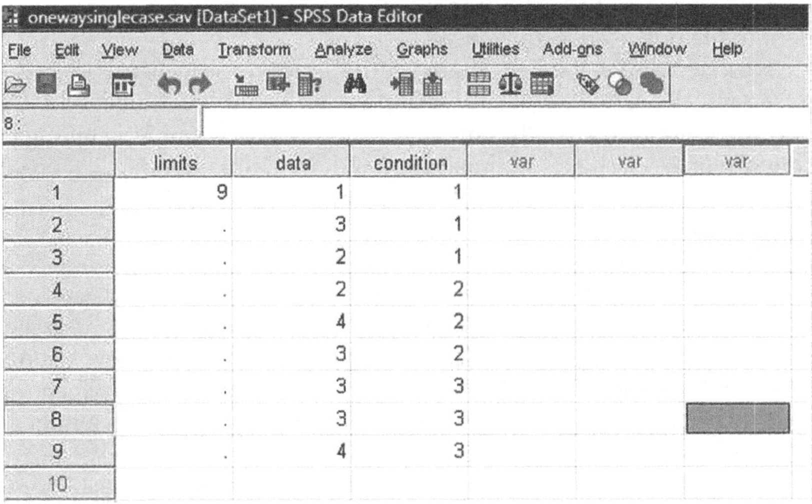

	limits	data	condition	var	var	var
1	9	1	1			
2	.	3	1			
3	.	2	1			
4	.	2	2			
5	.	4	2			
6	.	3	2			
7	.	3	3			
8	.	3	3			
9	.	4	3			
10						

Figure 4.1a Datasheet for one-way single case design as seen in SPSS.

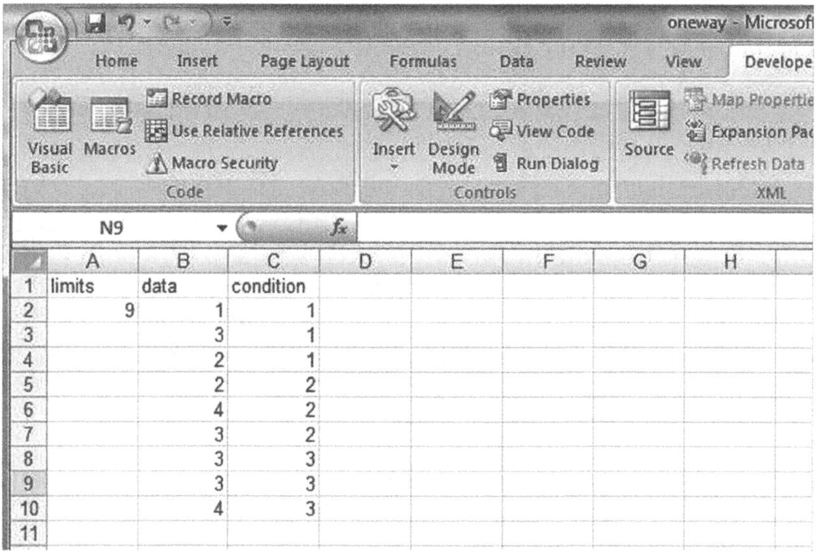

	A	B	C	D	E	F	G	H
1	limits	data	condition					
2	9	1	1					
3		3	1					
4		2	1					
5		2	2					
6		4	2					
7		3	2					
8		3	3					
9		3	3					
10		4	3					
11								

Figure 4.1b Datasheet for one-way single case design as seen in Excel.

(as used in ANOVA) will do that. In fact, we can either use *F*, which will be larger for greater differences among the condition means, or use the residual sum of squares (RSS) from the one-way ANOVA, which will be smaller for greater differences among the condition means. It's more convenient to calculate the RSS, so that is what we use. This means that we want to know whether the test statistic from the actual experiment is one of the smallest in the reference set.

Obtaining the reference set

The null hypothesis is that the number of activities our participant joins in is not affected by the three conditions. If this is true, then the condition labels are just arbitrary labels; and if we rearrange them and recalculate the test statistic, the only difference will be due to random variation. So we obtain the reference set by rearranging the labels and calculating the test statistic for each rearrangement.

It would be possible (though tedious and time consuming) to obtain the reference set by listing all possible arrangements, but the method used by our macro is the same as that used for all the designs in the book. We take 2000 random samples with replacement from the reference set, and this gives a good estimate of where the test statistic from the actual experiment lies. These two methods of obtaining the reference set are explained near the end of Chapter 2.

The analyses using SPSS and Excel are presented in Chapter 5, along with the analyses for the examples in the rest of this chapter.

A small-n one-way design

Our example

Suppose we want to know whether four different communication aids (think of Stephen Hawking and his speech synthesizer as one example) that are designed for people who are unable to speak differ in the time it takes to learn to use them to some criterion. We have 10 participants who are willing to try any of them. We also have two each of two of the aids and three each of the other two. We will record the number of hours of practice needed to reach the criterion.

Decisions to make

Before we can implement this design, we need to decide the following:

1. How many conditions (here we have four, the types of communication aid)
2. How many participants (here we have 10)
3. The numbers of participants to be allocated to each condition, which need not be equal (here the numbers of aids available mean we will allocate to 2, 2, 3, and 3 participants to the four types of aid)

We need to be confident that our participants are similar. If they are not, then a repeated-measures design may be considered instead.

Calculating the number of possible arrangements

With 10 participants assigned to four types of aid with 2, 2, 3, and 3 of each type of aid respectively, we have a total of $10!/(2!2!3!3!)$ or 25,200 possible arrangements. However, as in the single-case example, we have to allow for the fact that rearranging the condition labels for equal-sized groups would not alter the test statistic. There are two groups of size 2, and if we swap their condition labels the test statistic will not change, so we have two ways to arrange the labels for these two conditions, leaving 25,200/2 or 12,600 possible arrangements. There are also two groups of size 3, and if we swap their condition labels the test statistic will not change, so we have two ways to arrange the labels for these two conditions, leaving 12,600/2 or 6300 possible arrangements with distinct test statistics. This is certainly plenty to give us the possibility of a significant result.

Performing the randomization

Any method of randomization that gives the correct numbers in the four groups will do. Number the types of aid 1, 2, 3, and 4 (we are assuming we have two each of types 1 and 2, and three each of types 3 and 4). A quick way to do the randomization is to use SPSS or Excel to arrange the numbers 1, 1, 2, 2, 3, 3, 3, 4, 4, and 4 in random order as shown in Appendix 1. Number the participants according to date of birth or in some other way, and then use the random order of types of aid to assign the aids to the participants.

The datasheet

Once the participants have each been assigned an aid, collect the data and record in the SPSS or Excel datasheet as shown in Table 4.2, remembering to retain our variable names. The number in column 1 is the number of observations.

The test statistic

As for the single case, we use the RSS as our test statistic, so we shall want to know whether the RSS from the actual experiment is in the smallest 5% of the reference set.

Obtaining the reference set

The null hypothesis is that the time taken by our participants to learn to use the communication aids does not depend on the type of aid. If this is true, then the condition labels are just arbitrary labels; and if we rearrange them and recalculate the test statistic, the only difference will be

Table 4.2 Datasheet for
One-Way Small-n Design

Limits	Data	Condition
10	4	1
	4	1
	2	2
	4	2
	5	3
	4	3
	5	3
	7	4
	6	4
	6	4

due to random variation. So we obtain the reference set by rearranging the labels and calculating the test statistic for each rearrangement. As for the single-case and indeed all designs in this book, the macro takes a random sample with replacement of 2000 arrangements from the reference set. The analysis is presented in Chapter 5.

A small-n one-way design with two conditions

Our example

We want to find out whether doing active play reduces problem behavior in a subsequent learning activity in children with learning disabilities. We will compare active play with passive play. Children can choose one of several available tasks in each condition so they get to do something they enjoy. The active play choices are run, do stretching exercises, or dance, and the passive play tasks are watch a cartoon, play a game on the computer, or listen to music. We will compare the active play with passive play. We have nine suitable children willing to participate. A therapist observer, who will not know which condition the children are assigned, will count the problem behaviors during a half-hour classroom session immediately following the play session.

Decisions to make

We can use this design only if there are just two conditions, so the only decisions are as follows:

1. How many participants (here we have nine)
2. The numbers of participants to be allocated to each condition, which need not be equal (we will assign five children to active play [condition 1] and four to the passive play [condition 2])

Calculating the number of possible arrangements

The number of possible arrangements is 9!/(5!4!) or 126. There are only two conditions, and our test statistic will allow a directional hypothesis (in fact, we shall use the difference between condition means). As we noted at the end of the introduction to this section, with only two conditions we do not need to consider rearrangements of the condition labels. We have enough to give us the possibility of a significant result.

Performing the randomization

Any method of randomization that assigns five children to condition 1 and four to condition 2 will do. If the children are arranged in a list, then we can use SPSS or Excel to arrange the numbers 1, 1, 1, 1, 1, 2, 2, 2, and 2

Table 4.3 Datasheet for One-Way Small-*n* Design With Only Two Conditions

Limits	Data	Condition
9	4	1
	4	1
	1	1
	2	1
	0	1
	4	2
	6	2
	2	2
	5	2

in random order (see Appendix 1) and assign the activities in the resulting order to the children.

The datasheet

Once the children are assigned to the play conditions, collect the data and arrange in the SPSS or Excel datasheet as in Table 4.3. The number in column 1 is the number of observations. Remember to use the same variable names as shown.

The test statistic

In this case, because we have only two conditions, we can use the difference between the condition means as our test statistic, and it is possible to have a directional alternative hypothesis. Our macro uses as the test statistic the condition 2 mean minus the condition 1 mean, $\bar{x}_2 - \bar{x}_1$. The null hypothesis is that the two conditions make no difference to our measurement. If a directional prediction is made, the alternative hypothesis is that condition 2 *increases* the measurement, and the codes 1 and 2 should be assigned to the conditions accordingly.

In our example, we hope the active play (condition 1) will *reduce* problem behavior, so our directional prediction is that the condition 1 mean will be smaller than condition 2. Our coding for the two conditions is correct for the macro, which will use $\bar{x}_2 - \bar{x}_1$ as the test statistic and count the number in the reference set at least as large as our actual one. If we were counting desirable behaviors and predicting that the active play would increase them, it would be necessary to code the passive play as condition 1 (predicted smaller mean) and the active play as condition 2 (predicted larger mean).

Obtaining the reference set

If the null hypothesis is true, then the condition labels are just arbitrary labels, and rearranging them will only alter the test statistic by random variation. As usual, we take a random sample with a replacement of 2000 rearrangements and find the test statistic for each.

For the directional alternative hypothesis, we use a one-tailed test and find how many of the reference set values are at least as large as the one from the actual experiment. If the alternative hypothesis is that there is a difference between the conditions but we cannot predict in which direction, we use a two-tailed test and count reference set statistics that are at least as big as our actual one on either side of zero, as we would for a two-tailed *t* test. The macro does the work, and as you will see when the analysis is presented in Chapter 5 we just choose the appropriate test result.

A single-case randomized blocks design

The analysis of the single-case randomized blocks design is the same as that for the small-*n* repeated-measures design (the next example); only the experimental context is different. With the single-case randomized blocks design, we take measurements on our single participant in two or more conditions and we repeat the full set of measurements in at least two blocks of time. In each block of time, the conditions are applied in random order.

Our example

We have a neuropsychology patient who doesn't do his prescribed hourly relaxation exercises, even though he can remember them. We can give him a pager that will prompt him. Will a single prompt get him to do it, or would two be more effective? He is more motivated on some days than others to do the exercises, so we need to allow for this in the design. Allowing for breaks for lunch and dinner, we can divide each day into three 4-hour sessions with one type of prompt used in each session. He should do his exercises four times in each session, once every hour. For each session his partner will record the number of times (out of four) that he does the exercises. The null hypothesis is that the number of prompts given has no effect on the number of times he does the exercises.

Decisions to make

For this design, we need to decide the following:

1. How many conditions (three here: no prompt, a single prompt, and two prompts)

2. What makes a block (a day here, because the response may vary from day to day)
3. How to divide up a block into observation occasions, with the same number of occasions in each block as there are conditions (we can have three sessions in each block)
4. How many blocks (we will use three)

The conditions must be assigned in random order within each block, with each condition occurring once in each block. Here one 4-hour session counts as one block.

Calculating the number of possible arrangements

There are 3! or 6 ways to arrange the three conditions on the first day. Any of these can be paired with any of the 6 ways to arrange the conditions on the second day, giving 6*6 or 36 arrangements for the first 2 days. Any of these can be combined with any of the 6 ways to arrange conditions on the third day, so we have 36*6 or 216 arrangements. However, we have more than two conditions and the test statistic will treat all conditions in the same way (as noted in the introduction to this section), so rearranging the condition labels among equal-sized groups would not alter the test statistic. Our three groups are the same size, and there are 3! or 6 ways to arrange three conditions, so our 216 arrangements will only give 216/6 or 36 different test statistics. This is still enough to make a significant result a possibility.

Performing the randomization

Any randomization method that assigns the three conditions in random order on each day will do. Label the conditions 1, 2, and 3 and rearrange the numbers 1, 2, and 3 in random order using SPSS or Excel. Repeat the randomization two more times for days 2 and 3.

The datasheet

Once the conditions are assigned in random order to each day, collect the data and arrange in the SPSS or Excel datasheet as in Table 4.4. The first number in column 1 is the total number of observations (nine in this example, three on each of three days). The second number in column 1 is the number of blocks (3 days in this example). Remember to retain the variable names.

The test statistic

Just as in the one-way design, we need a test statistic that enables us to compare more than two conditions. We use the RSS again, for the same reasons as before.

Table 4.4 Datasheet for Single-Case
Randomized Blocks Design

Limits	Data	Condition	Block
9	0	1	1
3	2	2	1
	3	3	1
	1	1	2
	1	2	2
	4	3	2
	0	1	3
	2	2	3
	3	3	3

Obtaining the reference set

If the null hypothesis is true and the conditions have no effect on the number of times he does the exercises, the condition labels are just arbitrary labels, and rearranging them will only alter the test statistic by random variation. The rearrangements must conform to the design, in this case retaining each condition once in each block. So within each block, the condition labels are rearranged and the test statistic recalculated. As usual, we take a random sample with a replacement of 2000 rearrangements to estimate where our actual statistic falls in the reference set.

A small-n repeated-measures design

Our example

We could use a small-group repeated-measures design to test the effectiveness of pager prompts in getting patients to do their prescribed exercises. This time, instead of using a single case as described in the last example, we suppose we have four similar patients willing to participate for one day. Each participant will have the day divided into three 4-hour sessions and will receive each of the three conditions (no prompt, single prompt, and two prompts) once. The order in which the conditions are received is randomly selected for each participant. The exercises should be done four times, once per hour, during a session, and participants' partners will report the number of times out of four the exercises were completed for each condition. In this design, the participants replace the blocks from the previous design.

In this and the previous example, we have described a problem where we could use either a single-case or a small-*n* design. The single-case version would be appropriate if we wanted to find a solution for a particular patient. The small-group version in this section would be more useful if we hoped to find a strategy that would help patients of a particular type or if limited time per patient is available for the study. So, assuming we have several similar patients with a similar problem doing the prescribed exercises, we could include all those willing to be in our experiment.

Decisions to make

For this design, we need to decide the following:

1. How many conditions (three here: no prompt, a single prompt, and two prompts)
2. How many participants (we have four)

Each participant must receive each condition once (these are the repeated measures), and they must be applied in random order.

Calculating the number of possible arrangements

There are 3! or 6 ways to arrange 3 conditions in order. Any order can be used for any participant, so there are 6*6*6*6 or 1296 arrangements. However, as in the randomized blocks design, not all of them will give different test statistics. Any rearrangement of the condition labels among themselves will give the same test statistic. There are 3! or 6 ways to arrange the 3 condition labels so 1296/6 or 216 of our possible arrangements will give distinct test statistics. This is plenty to allow the possibility of a significant result.

Performing the randomization

Number the participants by date of birth or in some other way. Number the conditions 1, 2, and 3, then get SPSS or Excel to arrange the numbers 1, 2, and 3 in random order. This is the order for the first participant. Rearrange in random order three more times for the other participants.

The datasheet

Once the conditions have been assigned in random order to participants, arrange the data in the SPSS or Excel datasheet as in Table 4.5. The first number in the LIMITS column is the total number of observations, and the second is the number of participants (blocks).

The test statistic

The test statistic is the RSS exactly as in the randomized blocks design, and the analysis is the same with participants acting as the blocks in this case.

Table 4.5 Datasheet for Small-Group
Repeated-Measures Design

Limits	Data	Condition	Block
12	0	1	1
4	1	2	1
	3	3	1
	1	1	2
	2	2	2
	4	3	2
	1	1	3
	1	2	3
	3	3	3
	0	1	4
	2	2	4
	4	3	4

Obtaining the reference set

Just as in the last example, we take a random sample with a replacement of 2000 rearrangements of conditions within participants. If the null hypothesis is true and the conditions make no difference to the number of times exercises are done, the test statistics from the rearrangements will only differ by random variation.

A single-case randomized blocks design with two conditions

As in the one-way design, when we have only two conditions to test, a directional alternative hypothesis with a one-tailed test is possible. Once again we provide an extra macro for this special case. We illustrate it with a single case example, but it can also be used for a small-*n* repeated-measures design with just two conditions.

Our example

Staff at a pain clinic suspect that a new painkiller (A) will give longer relief to a cancer patient than their standard one (B). The patient is willing to try them in turn for several days, and record the number of hours before she needs another painkiller. The tablets can be made to look alike, and a set of test tablets can be made up in a strip to be taken in order. Some days are worse than others, so each day will have to be a block, and once each in the morning and afternoon when a painkiller is needed the patient will use one from the test strip and record the time to the next painkiller. Apart from these test occasions, the patient will take her usual painkiller.

Decisions to make

Because there are only two conditions, the only decisions to make are as follows:

1. What constitutes a block (a day here)
2. How many blocks we can use

Let us suppose the patient is willing to try this for a working week. So each test drug must be taken once each day, in random order, for 5 days.

Calculating the number of possible arrangements

For each day, there are two possible arrangements so we have a total of 2*2*2*2*2 or 32 arrangements. This does give the possibility of a result significant at 5%, but only using a one-tailed test and only if the actual result is the most extreme in the reference set, because 1/32 is 3% but 2/32 is 6%. As in other designs with only two conditions, we do not need to consider rearrangements of the condition labels.

Performing the randomization

Toss a coin or use SPSS or Excel to decide whether drug A or B is first on day 1. Then repeat for the other 4 days. The test strip of tablets will then be made up with A and B in the correct order for the whole 5 days.

The datasheet

Once the drugs are assigned in random order for each day, collect the data and arrange in the SPSS or Excel worksheet as in Table 4.6. In the LIMITS column, we have the number of blocks (or participants). If a one-tailed test

Table 4.6 Datasheet for Single-Case Randomized Blocks Design With Two Conditions

Limits	Data	Condition	Block
5	4	1	1
	5	2	1
	3	1	2
	5	2	2
	3	1	3
	4	2	3
	2	1	4
	4	2	4
	3	1	5
	5	2	5

with a directional alternative hypothesis is to be used, code the condition predicted to give the higher mean as 2. In our case, we record the length of time to the next painkiller, and we predict drug A will have the higher value so drug A is coded 2 and the standard drug B is coded 1.

The test statistic

With only two conditions to test, we can use the difference between condition means as our test statistic, and it is possible to have a directional alternative hypothesis. Our macro uses as the test statistic the condition 2 mean minus the condition 1 mean, $\bar{x}_2 - \bar{x}_1$. The null hypothesis is that the two conditions make no difference to our measurement. If a directional prediction is made, the alternative hypothesis is that condition 2 *increases* the measurement, and the codes 1 and 2 should be assigned to the conditions accordingly. We have assigned code 2 to drug A, predicted to give a longer period of relief than the standard drug B.

Obtaining the reference set

As usual, we take a random sample with replacement of 2000 rearrangements from the reference set. In this case, this means that the order of the two drugs is randomly assigned in each of the five blocks.

This is a case where listing the complete reference set would be possible, but we adopt a consistent approach and always estimate the position of our actual test statistic in the reference set by random sampling, as explained in Chapter 2.

A small-n repeated-measures design with two conditions and replicates

The macro for this design can be used in two ways, just as we use one macro for the single-case randomized blocks design and the small-*n* repeated-measures design. In the small-*n* repeated-measures design with two conditions described above, each participant receives each of the two conditions once. In the small-*n* repeated-measures design with two conditions and replicates described here, each participant receives each of the two conditions on several occasions. These repeat observations on each condition are the replicates.

The macro can also be used for a randomized blocks design with two conditions, but with several observations on each condition (the replicates) in each block. To use the macro in this way, we have blocks instead of participants. We make several observations in each condition in each block. We need a participant for each observation in this version of the design, so each participant appears in one block only and receives one condition from which we make a single observation. An example of this use of the design is provided in the exercises at the end of the chapter (questions 2 and 6).

Our example

We want to compare the efficiency of two pictorial depth cues: linear perspective and texture gradient. We show our participants two types of visual stimuli, one with the perspective cue and the other with the texture cue, and ask them to tell us how much depth they perceive in each (in centimeters). The two types of stimuli are presented twice each in random order for each participant. So if we indicate one as P (perspective) and the other T (texture), a random presentation sequence for one participant might look like this: PTTP. We have three volunteers for our experiment, and all of them are tested on both conditions in this way.

Decisions to make

For this design, we need to decide the following:

1. How many participants (we will have three)
2. How many observations on each condition for each participant (we will have two each of P and T)

Each participant must receive each condition the same number of times, and they must be applied in random order.

Calculating the number of possible arrangements

There are 4!/(2!2!) or 6 ways to arrange four picture cues, two each of P and T. Because we have three participants and each can receive the lists in any of the six orders, we have 6*6*6 or 216 possible arrangements, enough to give the possibility of a significant result. There are only two conditions, so as usual we do not need to consider rearrangements of condition labels.

Performing the randomization

Number the conditions 1 and 2, then use SPSS or Excel to arrange 1, 1, 2, and 2 in random order. This is the order for the first participant. Repeat for the other participants in turn.

The datasheet

Once the conditions have been assigned in random order to participants, collect the observations and arrange the data in the SPSS or Excel datasheet as in Table 4.7. The first number in the LIMITS column is the number of participants, and the second is the number of observations per participant.

Table 4.7 Datasheet for Small-*n* Repeated-
Measures Design With Replicates

Limits	Data	Condition	Participant
3	2	1	1
4	3	1	1
	4	2	1
	3	2	1
	4	1	2
	5	1	2
	7	2	2
	6	2	2
	2	1	3
	5	1	3
	4	2	3
	5	2	3

Because we have only two conditions, a directional hypothesis and a one-tailed test are possible. Our macro assumes that if we want to use this option, then the condition coded 2 would be expected to have the higher scores.

The test statistic

Because we have only two conditions, we can use the difference between condition means as the test statistic. If there is any difference between the efficiency of the type of pictorial depth cue, we would expect the perspective type (P) to result in greater depth perception, so we coded P as 2.

Obtaining the reference set

We take a random sample with replacement of 2000 rearrangements of conditions within participants. If the null hypothesis is true and the conditions make no difference to the perceived depth, the test statistics from the rearrangements will differ only by random variation.

A two-way factorial single-case design

Our example

A psychologist is trying to help a boy with attention deficit-hyperactivity disorder (ADHD) and his family. There are many problems, but this study will focus on his disturbed sleep. The psychologist thinks that both too much stimulation and junk food with sugar and additives make the problem worse, so she is investigating two factors each at two levels. Factor 1 is TV in his bedroom (banned or allowed), and factor 2 is junk food (banned or allowed). We will count the times he gets out of bed after he retires for the night. A camera in his room will film from bedtime until morning, and the psychologist will do the count so that results will not be biased by parental expectations or exhaustion. The four conditions are as follows:

TV and junk food both banned
TV banned and junk food allowed
TV allowed and junk food banned
TV and junk food both allowed

One of the conditions will be applied for the whole of each day in the experiment, and the count of disturbances will be made for the following night. The null hypotheses are that neither factor has any effect, and the alternatives are that banning TV or banning junk food will reduce the disturbance count.

Decisions to make
We can only use this design if we have two factors each at two levels, so there are only two decisions to make:

1. The number of observation occasions (we need a multiple of four so that we can get equal numbers in the four conditions)
2. The coding for the levels of the two factors because we want to use a directional alternative

Some nights are worse than others, so there will be some random variation even if the factors have no effect. The psychologist, the family, and the boy agree that 16 days and the following nights will be used for the experiment.

Because we want to use directional alternatives and one-tailed tests, we will code TV allowed as 2 for factor 1 and junk food allowed as 2 for factor 2, because these are the levels predicted to give higher counts.

Calculating the number of possible arrangements
Consider the main effect of junk food first. (For the main effect of TV, we just reverse the roles of junk food and TV in this and the following paragraph.) To find the main effect of junk food (allowed or disallowed), we need to consider the possible rearrangements of the levels of junk food (allowed, coded 2; and disallowed, coded 1). Because our design needs equal numbers of observations in all conditions, the levels of junk food can be rearranged only within TV allowed and within TV disallowed.

For the 8 days with TV allowed, we can arrange the 4 junk food–allowed days and the 4 junk food–disallowed days in $8!/(4!4!)$ or 70 ways. Also for the TV disallowed condition, we can arrange the four junk food–allowed and four junk food–disallowed days in 8!/(4!4!) or 70 ways. Any of the TV allowed arrangements can be combined with any TV disallowed arrangement, giving us 70*70 or 4900 altogether, certainly enough to give us the possibility of a significant result for the main effect of junk food. The factors have only two conditions, so as usual we do not need to consider rearrangements of their labels.

Performing the randomization
Any method of randomization that assigns 4 days to each of the four conditions will do. One method would be to number the conditions 1 to 4 and enter 1, 1, 1, 1, 2, 2, 2, 2, 3, 3, 3, 3, 4, 4, 4, and 4 into the SPSS or Excel datasheet and rearrange them in random order as shown in Appendix 1. Then apply the conditions to the test days in that order.

The datasheet
Once conditions are randomly assigned to test days, collect the data and enter into the SPSS or Excel datasheet as shown in Table 4.8, remembering that level 2 is allowing TV for factor 1 and allowing junk food for factor 2. The first column, LIMITS, gives the total number of observations, which must be a multiple of 4.

Table 4.8 Datasheet for Two-Way Factorial Single-Case Design

Limits	Data	Factor1	Factor2
16	1	1	1
	0	1	1
	3	1	1
	1	1	1
	3	1	2
	3	1	2
	2	1	2
	6	1	2
	3	2	1
	7	2	1
	8	2	1
	8	2	1
	9	2	2
	5	2	2
	4	2	2
	6	2	2

The test statistic

Factor 1 has just two levels, so we can use the difference between means as the test statistic for the main effect. Our macro uses the level 2 mean minus the level 1 mean, $\bar{x}_2 - \bar{x}_1$. For the one-tailed test of the alternative that level 2 (TV allowed) of the factor results in more disturbances, we count the values in the reference set that are at least as large as our actual value.

Factor 2 also has two levels, so we again use the difference between means as our test statistic. Once again, level 2 (junk food allowed) is predicted to have the higher mean, and we count values in the reference set at least as large as ours.

Obtaining the reference set

The null hypothesis for the main effect of factor 1 is that there is no difference between allowing TV and banning it. If this is true, then the level labels are just arbitrary labels and can be rearranged within each level of factor 2, and the test statistics will only be changed by random variation. As usual, our macro takes a random sample with replacement of 2000 such arrangements to get the main effect of factor 1, TV allowed or not.

For the main effect of factor 2, junk food allowed or not, we rearrange the factor 2 level labels within TV allowed and within TV banned. We shall use a one-tailed test for each main effect because we have directional alternatives for both (TV allowed results in more disturbances, and junk food allowed results in more disturbances). So in each case, we shall need to know how many values in the reference set are at least as large as our actual one.

A two-way factorial small-n design

Our example

We now extend our example for the one-way design with just two conditions. We wanted to test whether active play would reduce problem behavior in learning-disabled children. Our two conditions were active or passive play, and in both conditions the child was playing alone. Now we suppose that we also want to see whether there is any difference in outcome when the children are in a group. So we have two factors each at two levels (play active or passive, and alone or in a group). The four conditions are as follows:

Active play alone
Active play in a group
Passive play alone
Passive play in a group

To use our macro, we need the same number of observations in each of the four conditions.

Decisions to make

We can only use this design if we have two factors each at two levels, so there are only two decisions to make:

1. The number of participants (we need a multiple of four, so that we can get equal numbers in the four conditions)
2. The coding for the levels of the two factors because we want to use a directional alternative

Let's suppose 16 children are willing to participate, so we can assign four to each condition.

If a directional alternative hypothesis with a one-tailed test is to be used, then our macro assumes that level 2 of a factor is predicted to have the higher mean. For factor 1, we must code the passive play as 2 because we expect the passive play to result in more problem behavior than the active play. The coding for factor 2 (alone or in a group) is arbitrary because we do not predict the direction of the difference if there is one. We will use code 1 for alone and 2 for in a group.

Calculating the number of possible arrangements

First consider the main effect of play (active, coded 1; or passive, coded 2). To get the main effect of play, we need the possible rearrangements of the play levels (active or passive). Because of the requirement for equal numbers in each condition, the play levels can only be rearranged within play alone and within play in a group.

Within the 8 children playing alone, we can rearrange the four play 1s (active) and four play 2s (passive), giving $8!/(4!4!)$ or 70 arrangements. We can also rearrange the four play 1s and four play 2s for the 8 children playing in a group, giving another 70 arrangements. Any arrangement from the first 70 can be paired with any from the second 70, giving $70*70$ or 4900 altogether. This will certainly suffice to allow us the possibility of a significant result for the main effect of play (active or passive). Even if we look at the simple effects (the effect of active or passive play within playing alone for instance), we still have 70 arrangements, so significance is possible. Similar calculations apply to the main effect of alone or in a group, and to the simple effects of this factor. Even though we want to use a two-tailed test for alone or in a group, because 2/70 is only 0.03 we still have the possibility of obtaining a result significant at the 5% level.

Table 4.9 Datasheet for Two-Way
Factorial Small-*n* Design

Limits	Data	Factor1	Factor2
16	4	1	1
	4	1	1
	1	1	1
	2	1	1
	0	1	2
	3	1	2
	3	1	2
	3	1	2
	4	2	1
	6	2	1
	2	2	1
	5	2	1
	8	2	2
	6	2	2
	6	2	2
	5	2	2

Performing the randomization

Any method of randomization that assigns four children to each condition will do. List the children by date of birth or in some other way, and number the conditions 1 to 4. Then use SPSS or Excel to arrange four 1s, four 2s, four 3s, and four 4s in random order and apply the conditions to the children in this random order.

The datasheet

Once the children are randomly assigned to conditions, collect the data and arrange in the SPSS or Excel datasheet as shown in Table 4.9, using the same variable names. In the LIMITS column, we have the total number of observations, which must be a multiple of four.

The test statistic

Because we have just two levels for each factor, we can use the difference between level means as the test statistic for the main effects. Our macro uses the level 2 mean minus the level 1 mean, $\bar{x}_2 - \bar{x}_1$. For the one-tailed test of the alternative hypothesis that level 2 of the factor results in more problem behavior, we count the values in the reference set that are at least as large as our actual value. For the two-tailed test, the sign of the difference is ignored both for the actual test statistic and those in the reference set.

If we want to look at simple effects we use the macro *onewaytwoconditions*. For instance, if we want the simple effect of type of play within playing alone, just take the data for playing alone and use it in *onewaytwoconditions* with the codes for the two play types in the condition column.

Obtaining the reference set

The null hypothesis for the main effect of play type (factor 1) is that there is no difference between the active and passive play. If this is true, then the play labels are just arbitrary labels and can be rearranged within alone or in a group, and the test statistics will only be changed by random variation. As usual, our macro takes a random sample with replacement of 2000 such arrangements to get the main effect of factor 1.

For the main effect of factor 2, alone or in a group, we rearrange these labels within each play type. We shall use a two-tailed test for the main effect of factor 2 because we have made no directional alternative hypothesis.

Phase designs

All the macros for phase designs code the baseline phase as zero and the intervention phase as 1 in the datasheet. If there is a withdrawal phase, this is also coded as zero. Participants or measurements for the multiple baseline designs are numbered from 1.

To use directional hypotheses and one-tailed tests, the macros assume that the change predicted by the alternative hypothesis is for an *increase* in the measured variable. If the prediction is for a *decrease*, then the data must be transformed by subtracting them from a convenient number larger than any of them. This is illustrated in the example for the single-case AB design.

A single-case AB design

We will use as our example for the single-case AB design an intervention where withdrawal is impossible because any effect is likely to be permanent.

Our example

We are attempting to help a patient to cope with chronic pain, preferably without increasing the doses of painkiller to the point where functioning is impaired. We are going to try mindfulness training, which has been shown to help some people by enabling them to reduce the distress caused by their pain. Our data will be pain distress scores, collected each day during the trial.

Decisions to make

The decisions to make are as follows:

1. The total number of observations
2. The minimum number for the baseline phase
3. The minimum number for the intervention phase

Our patient is ready to use 35 days for the trial. There is bound to be some random variation from day to day, so we think we need at least 5 days in the baseline and at least 6 in the intervention phase. The intervention (the mindfulness training) will be given at the start of the first day of the intervention phase.

Calculating the number of possible arrangements

The intervention phase can begin on day 6, 7, 8, ... up to day 30, which is the last that will leave six for the intervention phase (days 30, 31, 32, 33, 34, and 35). This gives 25 possible intervention points, so if our test statistic is the largest, we shall have a result significant at the 5% level.

Performing the randomization

All we have to do is choose a random number between 6 and 30, and this will be the start day for the intervention. Appendix 1 shows how to choose a random number in a given range. When we did this for our example, we got number 8, so for us intervention starts on day 8.

The datasheet

If we want to use a directional alternative, as we do here, then the macro assumes that the intervention phase is predicted to have the larger mean. This is not the case for our example because the mindfulness training is designed to reduce the pain distress scores. If the prediction is for the intervention to reduce the mean, then the easiest way to set up the datasheet is to subtract all scores from some convenient round number that is larger than any of those obtained in the experiment. We illustrate this process using this example.

The distress scores obtained for the 35 days, in order, were 21, 36, 26, 17, 27, 28, 27, 9, 8, 21, 15, 13, 15, 13, 14, 17, 11, 15, 15, 13, 21, 27, 11, 10, 13, 20, 17, 21, 15, 13, 23, 11, 3, 18, and 17. You can see that the largest score is 36, so subtracting each score from any number at least as large as 36 would do the job. It's usually best to use a round number because that makes any subsequent checking easy, and we chose to use 50, but we could have used 100 or indeed 40.

So, once the data are obtained (and subtractions done if necessary), arrange them in three columns in the SPSS or Excel datasheet. In the first column, LIMITS, we have the total number of observations, then the

Table 4.10 Datasheet for Single-Case AB Design

Limits	Data	Phase	Data Cont	Phase Cont
35	29	0	35	1
5	14	0	37	1
6	24	0	29	1
	33	0	23	1
	23	0	39	1
	22	0	40	1
	23	0	37	1
	41	1	30	1
	42	1	33	1
	29	1	29	1
	35	1	35	1
	37	1	37	1
	35	1	27	1
	37	1	39	1
	36	1	47	1
	33	1	32	1
	39	1	33	1
	35	1		

minimum for baseline followed by the minimum for intervention. The second column, DATA, contains the observations, in this example the distress scores subtracted from 50 as explained above. The third column, PHASE, gives the phase for each observation with the baseline phase coded zero and the intervention phase coded 1. In Table 4.10 we have shown the example data with continuation columns for DATA and PHASE in order to make a compact table. The dataset is on the book Web site as *singlecaseAB. sav* (SPSS) and in the Excel workbook *singlecaseAB.xlsm*.

The test statistic

The test statistic will be the difference between the intervention (phase B) and baseline (phase A) means, $\bar{x}_B - \bar{x}_A$. The null hypothesis is that the intervention makes no difference. If the alternative is that it does make a difference but we do not predict in which direction, then we use a two-tailed test. Here our alternative is that the intervention results in an increase in the (transformed) scores, so we use a one-tailed test.

Obtaining the reference set

If the null hypothesis is true, then altering the point at which the phase label changes from 0 to 1 will make no difference except random variation.

To obtain the reference set, we only need to recalculate the test statistic as if the intervention point had been at each of the possible points from which we chose the actual one. In practice, to conform to the rest of our macros, we take a random sample with replacement of 2000 possible intervention points to estimate where in the reference set our actual test statistic falls.

A single-case ABA design

For this design, we use an example where the intervention is expected to increase the mean score, so the data can be used just as collected for this case. To see how to adjust an expected decrease in score, refer to the AB design.

Our example

A patient who suffered a head injury has difficulty linking subtasks together to complete a larger task. We hope to improve his ability to prepare his own breakfast and we have compiled a checklist, "take bowl from cupboard," "take milk from fridge," and so on. There are 10 items on the list, and his partner will count the number of stages accomplished each day for a successful breakfast. Baseline observations will be made before the list is introduced, then the list will be withdrawn for the withdrawal stage. We hope that using the list will increase the patient's scores, but we expect that the effect will not be maintained once the list is withdrawn. We can set aside 15 days for the study.

Decisions to make

The decisions to make are as follows:

1. The total number of observations
2. The minimum number for the baseline phase
3. The minimum number for the intervention phase
4. The minimum number for the withdrawal phase

We can use 15 days for the trial, and this will be the total number of observations. We believe we need a minimum of three each in the baseline and withdrawal phases, and four in the intervention phase.

Calculating the number of possible arrangements

Appendix 1 and the example of a single-case ABA design in Chapter 2 show the details of calculating the number of possible intervention–withdrawal pairs. Here, with three observations needed for baseline, the first possible intervention point would be day 4. If this is chosen, the first possible withdrawal day would be day 8 (allowing days 4, 5, 6, and 7 for intervention) and the last possible withdrawal day would be day 13 (allowing days 13, 14, and 15 for withdrawal). So with intervention on day 4, we have 6 possible withdrawal days. If intervention starts on day 5, withdrawal could not start until at least day 9 and would still be possible up to day 13, giving 5 possibilities. In a similar way we can have 4, 3, 2, and 1 possible withdrawal days if the intervention starts on day 6, 7, 8, and 9, respectively. Day 9, is the latest possible start for intervention because we need 4 days for intervention and 3 for withdrawal (days 9, 10, 11, and 12 and days 13, 14, and 15). So altogether we have 6 + 5 + 4 + 3 + 2 + 1 or 21 possible pairs of intervention and withdrawal points, which does allow the possibility of a result significant at the 5% level.

Performing the randomization

To perform the randomization, first list the possible intervention–withdrawal pairs. For this example, you can see the list in Table 4.11. (Appendix 1 shows how to do this in a systematic way using a different example.) Number the pairs from 1 (up to 21 in this case). Now choose a random number between 1 and 21 (for a different number of pairs, the range would be 1 to the number of pairs). Appendix 1 shows how to choose a random number in a given range. Now return to the numbered list of pairs to find the randomly chosen intervention and withdrawal points. Our random number between 1 and 21 was 14. In Table 4.11 you can see that this corresponds to the pair (6,12), so our intervention point is 6 and our withdrawal point is 12.

The datasheet

Our data are shown in Table 4.12. In the LIMITS column, we have the total number of observations, then the minimum for baseline, the minimum for intervention, and the minimum for withdrawal. The baseline and withdrawal phases are coded zero, and the intervention phase is coded 1. In the DATA column are the counts of subtasks performed.

Table 4.11 Intervention and Withdrawal Points for a
Single-Case ABA Design

Intervention–Withdrawal Pairs	Identification Numbers					
(4,8) (4,9) (4,10) (4,11) (4,12) (4,13)	1	2	3	4	5	6
(5,9) (5,10) (5,11) (5,12) (5,13)		7	8	9	10	11
(6,10) (6,11) (6,12) (6,13)			12	13	14	15
(7,11) (7,12) (7,13)				16	17	18
(8,12) (8,13)					19	20
(9,13)						21

Table 4.12 Datasheet for Single-Case ABA Design

Limits	Data	Phase
15	4	0
3	2	0
4	5	0
3	3	0
	4	0
	10	1
	5	1
	7	1
	5	1
	7	1
	10	1
	4	0
	0	0
	5	0
	3	0

The test statistic

We use the difference between the intervention mean and the mean of the baseline and withdrawal observations as our test statistic, $\bar{x}_B - \bar{x}_A$. Our alternative hypothesis is that the intervention will increase the scores, and this statistic will be increased if our alternative hypothesis is correct.

Obtaining the reference set

If the null hypothesis is true and the intervention has no effect, then the phase labels are meaningless and we could change them in any way consistent with the minimum number of observations required for baseline, intervention, and withdrawal phases, and we would only alter the test statistic by random variation. In practice, our macro takes 2000 random samples with replacement from the possible pairs of intervention and withdrawal points and calculates the test statistic for each to estimate where our result comes in the reference set.

A multiple baseline AB design

This design is usually used with several participants. However, it may be used with a single participant if we want to test the effectiveness of several interventions during a single series of observation occasions. Here is an example with a single participant, but this same macro could be used with multiple participants rather than multiple measurements. For the multiple baseline ABA design, we have an example with several participants.

Our example

Our participant is a user of a communication aid (think of Stephen Hawking and his speech synthesizer). We want to test whether training in the use of "turn-around" questions that turn the conversation from talking about the user to talking about the partner (e.g., "What about you?" and "And you?") will lead to him being perceived as more competent as a conversational partner. We also want to test whether training in the use of feedback remarks that show that the user is paying attention to the partner (e.g., "I see," "Sure," and "Right") will lead to him being perceived as more interested. We have a conversational partner who is willing to be videoed in a series of short conversations with our participant. We also have two raters willing to watch the videos and rate our participant on how competent and how interested he seems. We can randomize separately the two points at which training is given in the use of turn-around questions and in the use of feedback remarks. From each observation occasion, two measurements are taken (the scores from the two raters). With this variant of the design, it is important that a different measurement is associated with each of the interventions. The two training interventions and the two series of measurements are analogous to an AB design with two participants so we can use the same macro. In this latter design, the intervention for each participant is selected separately, whereas in the present design, the intervention point for each training intervention is selected separately.

Decisions to make

If we are using this design with a single participant, then we need to decide the following:

1. How many observation occasions
2. How many measurements on each occasion
3. The minimum number for baseline (which must be the same for all measurements)
4. The minimum number for intervention (which must be the same for all measurements)

To use the design with several participants, taking a single measurement from each on each occasion, then in place of 2 above we must decide on how many participants. The minima for baseline and intervention must be the same for all participants.

For our example, we shall take two measurements on each occasion, and our participant and his partner are willing to do 15 observation occasions, one each weekday for three weeks. We think a minimum of four each in the baseline and intervention phases will suffice.

Calculating the number of possible arrangements

We can think of each measurement as having its own series of observation occasions. Because we need a minimum of four observations for baseline, the first possible day to start the intervention observations would be day 5. With 15 occasions the last day for starting the intervention would be day 12, leaving days 12, 13, 14, and 15 for intervention. This gives us eight possible choices for the start of intervention. With any of these eight, we could pair any of the eight possibilities for the other intervention, giving 8*8 or 64 possible pairs of intervention points for the two measurements. This is sufficient to allow the possibility of a result significant at the 5% level.

Performing the randomization

All we need to do is choose a random number between 5 and 12 (see Appendix 1 if you don't know how to do this) for the start of intervention for the first measurement. Then choose another random number in the same range for the start of intervention for the second measurement. Our random numbers were 6 (turn-around questions) and 8 (feedback remarks).

If we have several participants, choose a random number in the correct range for each participant to start intervention.

The datasheet

Once the intervention points are chosen at random, collect the data and arrange in four columns in the SPSS or Excel datasheet. The first column, LIMITS, contains the number of participants (or in our example, measurements) at the top, then the number of observation occasions for each participant (or measurement), then the minimum for baseline, and last the minimum for intervention.

In the second column, DATA, we have all the observations for the first participant or measurement, baseline followed by intervention, then the same for the next participant or measurement, and so on until all the data are entered. In the third column, PHASE, as usual baseline is coded as zero and intervention is coded as 1. In the fourth column, PARTICIPANT, we have the codes for the participants or measurements (they are numbered from 1). In Table 4.13 we have continuation columns for DATA, PHASE, and PARTICIPANT in order to make a compact table. The dataset can be found on the book Web site as *multiplebaselineAB.sav* (SPSS) or in the Excel workbook *multiplebaseline.xlsm*.

Table 4.13 Datasheet for Multiple Baseline AB Design

Limits	Data	Phase	Participant	Data Cont	Phase Cont	Participant Cont
2	5	0	1	4	0	2
15	4	0	1	5	0	2
4	5	0	1	3	0	2
4	3	0	1	3	0	2
	3	0	1	4	0	2
	6	1	1	3	0	2
	5	1	1	5	0	2
	5	1	1	7	1	2
	8	1	1	9	1	2
	4	1	1	9	1	2
	4	1	1	6	1	2
	5	1	1	8	1	2
	5	1	1	7	1	2
	5	1	1	7	1	2
	6	1	1	9	1	2

We will use a directional alternative hypothesis for each of our measurements (turn-around question training increases competence scores and feedback question training increases interest scores). Because in each case the direction predicts an increase, we can use the one-tailed test provided by the macro without transforming the data. If we had a directional alternative for only one measurement, then a one-tailed test could not be used because the two measurements are combined in the test (see the discussion below).

The test statistic

The test statistic will be the sum over the participants or measurements of the difference between the intervention and baseline means. So we find the difference between means for the competence score just as in the single-case AB design, then repeat for the interest score, and add the two results.

If we find a significant result using the one-tailed test, this will tell us only that at least one participant or measurement showed a significant increase. If we find a significant result using the two-tailed test, this will tell us only that at least one participant or measurement showed a significant change. Note that a significant result does not say anything specifically about either participant (or measurement).

Obtaining the reference set

If the null hypotheses are both true, then the phase labels are just arbitrary labels and moving the intervention point labels will only change the difference in the means by random variation. The macro takes a random sample with replacement of 2000 pairs of intervention points and calculates the difference between intervention and baseline means for each, to estimate the position of our test statistic in the reference set.

A multiple baseline ABA design

We use several participants for our example of a multiple baseline ABA design. We could use several measurements with this design as in the multiple baseline AB design above. As for the other phase designs, our macro assumes that if a directional alternative hypothesis is used, it predicts an increase in the variable measured.

Our example

Here we will use a variant of our single-case ABA example. We have three volunteer head injury patients who all experience similar difficulties in linking subtasks together to complete a task successfully. With several participants, we can use fewer observations for each of them and so reach a conclusion more quickly. We will use the same checklist for the breakfast task as we used with the single case.

Decisions to make

If we are using this design with several participants, then we need to decide the following:

1. How many observation occasions for each participant (they must all be the same)
2. How many participants
3. The minimum number for baseline
4. The minimum number for intervention
5. The minimum number for withdrawal

To use the design with a single participant, taking several measurements each with its own intervention, then in place of 2 above we must decide on how many measurements. The minima for baseline, intervention, and withdrawal must be the same for all participants (or measurements).

We have three volunteers and can use 10 observation occasions for each. We believe we need a minimum of three observations each for baseline and intervention, and two for withdrawal.

Calculating the number of possible arrangements

We can consider the participants one at a time. For the first, the earliest intervention day is 4, and if this is chosen we could withdraw on day 7, 8, or 9 (see the single-case ABA design for an explanation of this process). If intervention starts on day 5, withdrawal could start on day 8 or 9. The last possible start of intervention is day 6, and if this is chosen withdrawal must start on day 9. So there are 3 + 2 + 1 or 6 possible pairs of intervention and withdrawal points for each participant. Any choice is possible for all participants, so we have 6*6*6 or 216 possible arrangements, plenty to allow the possibility of a significant result.

Performing the randomization

All we have to do is perform the randomization for the first participant in exactly the same way as for the single-case ABA design, then repeat the process for each of the other two. Begin by listing the possible intervention–withdrawal pairs as shown for single-case ABA design in Table 4.11 (Appendix 1 has an additional example). A random number in the correct range (1 to 6 here) must be chosen to identify the intervention–withdrawal pair for participant 1. Choose a new random number to identify the intervention–withdrawal pair for each of the other participants. When we performed the randomization we obtained the following intervention and withdrawal days for our three participants, 4 and 8, 5 and 9, and 5 and 8.

The datasheet

Once the randomization is done, collect the data and arrange it in four columns in the SPSS or Excel datasheet. In the first column, LIMITS, we have the number of participants, then the number of observations for each of them, then the minimum for baseline, the minimum for intervention, and the minimum for withdrawal. In the second column, DATA, we have all the observations for the first participant, baseline then intervention then withdrawal, followed by all the observations for the next participant, and so on for all the participants. In the third column, PHASE, the baseline and withdrawal phases are coded zero and the intervention phase is coded 1. In the fourth column, PARTICIPANTS, the participants (or measurements if these are used instead) are numbered from 1. In Table 4.14 we have shown the data with continuation columns for DATA, PHASE, and PARTICIPANT to make a compact table. The dataset can be found on the book Web site as *multiplebaselineABA. sav* (SPSS) or the Excel workbook *multiplebaselineABA.xlsm*.

Our alternative hypothesis is directional, so we shall use the one-tailed test. Because we predict that the checklist will increase the breakfast score we do not need to transform the data by subtraction. If the prediction is

Table 4.14 Datasheet for Multiple Baseline ABA Design

Limits	Data	Phase	Participant	Data Cont	Phase Cont	Participant Cont
3	3	0	1	10	1	2
10	1	0	1	8	1	2
3	1	0	1	8	1	2
3	10	1	1	1	0	2
2	8	1	1	2	0	2
	9	1	1	3	0	3
	9	1	1	4	0	3
	4	0	1	1	0	3
	1	0	1	4	0	3
	2	0	1	8	1	3
	1	0	2	8	1	3
	3	0	2	10	1	3
	1	0	2	4	0	3
	1	0	2	2	0	3
	9	1	2	3	0	3

for a decrease, refer to the AB design for an explanation of how to do the transformation to change the prediction to an increase as required by the macro.

The test statistic

We used the difference between the intervention mean and the mean of the baseline and withdrawal observations as our test statistic for the single-case ABA design, $\bar{x}_B - \bar{x}_A$. As for the multiple baseline AB design, we sum the test statistics obtained from each participant and use this as our multiple baseline test statistic.

Obtaining the reference set

If the null hypothesis is true and the intervention has no effect, then we could change the phase labels for each participant in any way consistent with the minima required for baseline, intervention, and withdrawal, and we shall only alter the test statistic by random variation. In practice, our macro takes 2000 random samples with replacement from the possible pairs of intervention and withdrawal points for each participant and calculates the test statistic for each to estimate where our result comes in the reference set.

A design to test order effects

In Chapter 2 we illustrated the design for order effects with an example where we predicted a partial ordering of the results. We thought students receiving method 3 training would perform best, those receiving method 2 would be next best, and those receiving method 1 would perform worst, but we did not attempt to order the students within the methods. For our example here, we will use an example where we predict a complete ordering. The macro and analysis apply equally well to a complete or a partial ordering.

Our example

The idea is to investigate how prejudice influences our judgments even when, in fact especially when, we are unaware of it. We have 15 student teachers who do not know the real purpose of the experiment, but all have agreed to arrange in order of merit five short pieces of writing by primary school pupils. We have chosen the five pieces to be as close as possible in their use of English, so they should be very difficult to arrange in order and informed judges should disagree about the correct order. Names will be attached to the written work, and we use a very familiar boy's name and four further boys' names with decreasing familiarity. The five names can be arranged in order in 5! or 120 ways, and we choose 15 of these arrangements at random. Each participant receives a set of the five written pieces with the names attached in one of these 15 ways. So the five pieces of work have the five names attached in 15 different random ways. We are not interested in the rankings assigned to the pieces of work, only in the rankings assigned to each of the names, and we calculate the mean rank for each of the names. The null hypothesis is that the mean ranks of the names are just random, but the alternative is that the mean ranks will put the names in this order: most familiar name, second most familiar name, third most familiar name, fourth most familiar name, and fifth most familiar name.

Decisions to make

To use this design to test for order effects, we need to decide the following:

1. How many items are to be ordered (five names in our example)
2. How the ordering is to be done (average 15 rankings in our example) and
3. How randomization can be used (names assigned at random to the pieces of writing here)

Calculating the number of possible arrangements

There are 5! or 120 ways to arrange the five names in order. Only one of these orders agrees with our alternative hypothesis. If that is the order we observe, then our result will be significant at the 5% level.

Performing the randomization

Here we need to make sure that our randomization method assigns the names in a way that will give us a random ordering if the null hypothesis is true. We have ensured this by making the pieces of work as difficult as possible to arrange in order of merit, and by assigning names to those pieces in random order. We number the pieces of work from 1 to 5, and because we have 15 volunteers, we select at random 15 of the possible orderings of the names to apply to the pieces of work. Then each volunteer gets one of the sets with names attached. We code the names from most to least familiar from 1 to 5. We ask the volunteers to rank the pieces of work from best (1) to worst (5).

The datasheet

For each name, we find the mean rank from the 15 ranks assigned by our participants. These appear in the second column of the datasheet, as shown in Table 4.15. The LIMITS column shows the number of items ranked, and the PREDICT column shows our predicted ranking.

Obtaining the reference set

If the null hypothesis is true, we cannot predict the ranks of the names, and our predictions are just a random assignment of the numbers 1 to 5. In this case, any rearrangement of our predicted ranks will only alter the test statistic by random variation. As usual, we use a random sample of 2000 rearrangements to estimate the position of our actual test statistic in the reference set.

Table 4.15 Datasheet for Order Effects Design

Limits	Data	Predict
5	1.63	1
	1.63	2
	2.73	3
	4.33	4
	4.67	5

Exercises

1. Anecdotal evidence suggests that the nesting success of terns may be improved if there is some provision for chicks to shelter from attacks by gulls. A nature reserve with a large lake has seven anchored rafts to provide nest sites for terns. Suggest a one-way design to find out whether providing shelter improves nesting success. Check that there are enough possible arrangements for significance at 5% to be a possibility.

2. We want to compare relaxation training and mindfulness training as methods of pain reduction, and we have two kinds of pain to consider: neurological pain and muscle pain. Our first idea was a two-way factorial design, but we soon identified a problem. What was the problem?

3. We are using a multiple baseline AB design with 4 participants. The minimum number of observations for baseline is 4 and the minimum for intervention is 6. What is the minimum number of observations per participant if significance at 5% is to be a possibility?

4. If we are to use a multiple baseline AB design with at most 10 observations per participant and a minimum of 3 each for baseline and intervention, how many participants are needed to allow for the possibility of significance at 5% using a one-tailed test?

5. An ecologist is planning a pilot for a large reforestation project where rabbits might damage the bark of unprotected trees. He wants to know whether planting the young trees in individual tubes or providing rabbit-proof fencing around groups of trees gets better results. If fencing is to be used, he needs to know what size groups to fence. He expects that the tubes are best, fencing around small groups (about 20 trees) is next best, and fencing around large groups (about 40 trees) is least effective. Unfortunately, this is in inverse order of the cost, so if tubes are to be used, he needs some supporting data. Suggest a design for him.

6. Can you suggest a design for the problem described in question 2? One possibility is to adapt the small-*n* repeated-measures design with two conditions and replicates. Describe how this could be done. (*Hint*: The two types of pain can be two blocks.)

7. We are planning a one-way small-*n* design to test four remedial programs for poor readers. We have 15 suitable volunteers, and we would like to include them all, though obviously this means the treatment groups cannot be all the same size. Number the remedial programs from 1 to 4, and describe two ways in which you could randomly assign them to the participants. Which method must be used if analysis is to be done with our macro?

chapter five

Analyzing the data
Using the macros

Introduction

This chapter shows you how to use the macros for each of the designs described in the previous two chapters. In case you haven't used macros before, Appendices 2 (SPSS) and 3 (Excel) demonstrate how to run and edit a macro in each of the packages. Also in the appendices, we have provided listings of the macros with comments, but you only need to read these long sections if you want to edit the macros or write new ones yourself. To use the macros as they are, the easiest way is to take them from the book Web site (http://www.researchmethodsarena.com/9780415886932) along with the example data used for illustration in this chapter and the previous one. You will probably want to run the macros with the example data yourself before applying them to your own data. We remind you that when you run the macros with our example data for yourself, although the actual test statistics will be the same, the counts of arrangement statistics at least as extreme are unlikely to be exactly the same as ours because we take a random sample from the reference set, as explained in Chapter 2. The corresponding probabilities also vary a bit from one run to another. The SPSS and Excel results shown below are those from our own runs. Sometimes we remind you they are sample runs and quote results for another run.

We have given the macros names that correspond to the designs. So, for example, the first macro is called *oneway* as it deals with a design analogous to one-way ANOVA. As in Chapter 4, we have provided separate examples for the one-way design with a single case and with a small group, but the macro is the same. The single-case randomized blocks design and the small-*n* repeated measures design also use the same macro (called *randomizedblocks*), and we have again provided examples of its use for each design. We also have single-case and small-*n* examples for the two-way factorial design, but there is only one macro (called *factorial*).

There is an extra macro for the special case of *oneway* with only two conditions, called *onewaytwoconditions*. There is also an extra macro for *randomizedblocks* when there are only two conditions, called *randomizedblockstwoconditions*.

For designs where one- and two-tailed probabilities are both possible, we obtain the two-tailed probability by comparing the absolute value of the actual test statistic with the absolute values of the rearrangement test statistics. If the actual test statistic is positive, then of course its absolute value is the same.

Users of phase designs may be surprised to find that the one- and two-tailed probabilities can be the same. This result is likely when the intervention has a large effect that is seen at every intervention observation. Our single-case AB design provides an example. The intervention can start at any point from 6 to 30, and you can easily check for yourself that the 25 pairs of means are as follows when we move the supposed start of intervention from point 6 through point 30:

24.6 and 34.3 (means of first 5 and last 30 observations), 24.2 and 34.6 (means of first 6 and last 29 observations), 24.0 and 35.0, 26.1 and 34.8, 27.9 and 34.5, 28.0 and 34.8, 28.6 and 34.8, 29.3 and 34.6, 29.8 and 34.5, 30.7 and 34.4, 30.7 and 34.4, 30.8 and 34.5, 31.3 and 34.3, 31.5 and 34.2, 31.7 and 34.2, 31.9 and 34.0, 31.8 and 34.4, 31.4 and 35.2, 31.7 and 34.9, 32.1 and 34.4, 32.3 and 34.2, 31.2 and 34.7, 32.2 and 34.9, 32.1 and 35.7, and 32.2 and 35.8 (means of the first 29 and last 6 observations).

In each pair the second mean is greater than the first, so the differences $\bar{x}_B - \bar{x}_A$ are all positive, so not only our test statistic but also every value in the reference set is positive. There are no extreme negative values (in fact, no negative values at all), so even if we disregard the direction of the difference, we find no extra extreme values to make the two-tailed probability larger than the one-tailed probability. We make no further comment when results like this occur later in the chapter.

Near the end of the section on each design, we show possible wording for a report of the statistical conclusion. We use "rearrangement statistics" rather than "reference set" in these short paragraphs because your readers may understand this term more readily. These short summaries of the conclusions assume that a full description of the design and the test statistic used has already been given.

We divide the rest of this chapter into two parts, for SPSS and Excel, so you only need to read the part for the package you use.

Analyses using the SPSS macros

Each SPSS macro is contained in a syntax file with the extension *sps*, for example the first macro is *oneway.sps*. The example data files have the extension *sav*, for example the data for the first example are in *onewaysinglecase*.

sav. To run the macros with your own data, just delete the example data and enter your own, but keep the variable names the same.

SPSS prints small numbers in standard form, so 0.014 would appear as 10^{-2} times 1.4. In common with most software, SPSS uses ** to denote a power, so 0.014 will look like this:

$$10**-2 \times 1.4$$

Analogs of ANOVA: a single-case one-way design

Open the data file *onewaysinglecase.sav* and the syntax file *oneway.sps*. In the syntax window, select **Run** on the menu bar and then **All** to run the macro. Refer to Appendix 2 if you are not sure about this.

In a few seconds, the results appear in the Output window (see Figure 5.1 *SPSS Output 5.1*). Remember that your own runs are unlikely to produce exactly the same counts and probabilities as ours, though the test statistics will be the same. The heading **Matrix** (not shown here) appears because the SPSS macros use the matrix language. Below the heading is a statement (not shown here) of the data file that was used for the analysis. Below the heading "RSS" (for residual sum of squares) is the test statistic calculated from our actual experiment (4.67 for our example). This is the same RSS we would get if we performed a one-way ANOVA on our data.

Next is the count of RSS values from the 2000 sample rearrangements that are at least as small as ours (738 in the example shown). So including the RSS from the actual experiment we have 739 values at least as small as ours out of 2001. So the probability of a value as extreme as our actual one occurring by chance is 739/2001 or 0.369 or 37%. This is shown below the heading "probability." This is not less than 5%, so we would not reject the null hypothesis: Our experiment does not provide evidence that any of

```
Run MATRIX procedure:

RSS
     4.666666667

count of arrangement RSS at least as small
     738

probability
     .3693153423

------ END MATRIX -----
```

Figure 5.1 *SPSS Output 5.1*. Result from a single-case one-way design.

our methods makes any difference to the number of activities the participant joins in. The **statistical conclusion** could be reported as follows.

> We had three methods to test to see whether we could increase the number of activities in which our patient with Alzheimer's disease joined. In a randomization test of the null hypothesis that our methods did not affect the number of activities he joined, 37% of a random sample of 2000 rearrangement statistics were at least as small as our experimental value. This does not approach significance at the 5% level, and we conclude that we do not have evidence that our methods affect the number of activities he joined in.

As we mentioned above, because we take a random sample of 2000 rearrangements of the condition labels, if we run the macro again we expect a slightly different number of RSS values at least as small as the actual one. On a rerun, we found 757 values at least as small as the actual one, giving a probability of 0.379.

To use the macro with your own data, just replace the example data in the data file with your own, but keep the variable names the same.

Analogs of ANOVA: a small-n one-way design

The analysis for a one-way design with a small group is exactly the same as for a single case, but the participants replace the measurement occasions. The macro is the same, and the results are displayed in exactly the same way as for the single case. Hence our treatment of this example will be quite brief.

Open the data file *onewaysmallgroup.sav* and the syntax file *oneway.sps*. Run the macro as before. In a few seconds the results appear in the Output window (see Figure 5.2 *SPSS Output 5.2*). The results are set out in exactly the same way as for the single case.

You can see that there were only 12 arrangements at least as small as the one obtained from the actual experiment, so our RSS is in the smallest 13/2001 or 0.6% of the reference set. SPSS prints the probability in standard form, with a power of 10 times a number between 1 and 10. In this example the probability is given as $10^{**}-3$ or 10^{-3} times 6.497. So the probability of a result this small if the null hypothesis is true is 0.006497 or 0.6%. The **statistical conclusion** could be reported as follows.

> In a randomization test of the hypothesis that different communication aids would take different lengths of time to learn to a criterion, only 0.6% of a random sample of 2000 rearrangement statistics were at least as small as our experimental value. This is much less than 5%, so we reject the null hypothesis of no difference among times taken to learn to use the aids. Our experiment supports the alternative hypothesis that the different types of communication aid take different lengths of time to learn.

```
Run MATRIX procedure:

RSS
    3.333333333

count of arrangement RSS at least as small
    12

probability
    10 ** -3    X
    6.496751624

------ END MATRIX -----
```

Figure 5.2 *SPSS Output 5.2.* Result from a small-*n* one-way design.

Because we take a random sample of 2000 rearrangements of the condition labels, if we run the macro again we expect a slightly different number of RSS values at least as small as the actual one. On a rerun, we found 13 or 0.7% of values at least as small as the actual one.

To use the macro with your own data, just replace the example data in the data file with your own, but keep the variable names the same.

Analogs of ANOVA: a small-n one-way design with two conditions

To analyze our example of a one-way design with just two conditions, open the data file *onewaytwoconditions.sav* and the syntax file *onewaytwoconditions. sps*, and run the macro exactly as before. In a few seconds, we find the results in the Output window as shown in Figure 5.3 *SPSS Output 5.3*.

We see that the difference between the condition means is 2.05 (the passive play mean is 4.25, and the active play mean is 2.20). In our first run, we found 183 rearrangements gave a difference at least as large. This is what we need for the one-tailed test. So the one-tailed probability is 184/2001 or 0.092, because 184 out of 2001 or 9.2% of the reference set is at least as large as the actual test statistic. The **statistical conclusion** could be reported as follows.

> In a randomization test of the prediction that active play reduces problem behavior in a subsequent learning activity in children with learning disabilities, 9.2% of the rearrangement statistics were at least as large as our experimental value. This is not less than 5%, so we do not reject the null hypothesis: Our experiment did not provide evidence that active play reduced problem behavior in a subsequent learning activity.

```
Run MATRIX procedure:

test statistic
   2.050000000

count of arrangement statistics at least as large
   183

one tail probability
   10 ** -2 . X
    9.195402299

count of arrangement statistics at least as large in abs value as abs(test)
   309

two tail probability
   .1549225387

------ END MATRIX -----
```

Figure 5.3 *SPSS Output 5.3.* Result from a small-*n* one-way design with just two conditions.

If we are using a two-tailed test for a nondirectional hypothesis, the signs are ignored for the actual statistic and for those in the reference set. There were 309 arrangements with a test statistic at least as large as ours ignoring the signs. So our test statistic is in the top $310/2001 = 15.5\%$, well above 5%. In general, the two-tailed test will give a higher proportion of the reference set at least as large as our actual value.

To use the macro with your own data, just replace our example data in the data file with yours, but keep the variable names the same.

Analogs of ANOVA: a single-case randomized blocks design

To analyze our randomized blocks example, open the data file *random-izedblocks.sav* and the syntax file *randomizedblocks.sps*, and run the macro as before. In a few seconds the result appears in the output window as shown in Figure 5.4 *SPSS Output 5.4.*

Our actual test statistic (the RSS) is 1.78, and 108 rearrangements gave a value at least as small. So our test statistic is in the smallest $109/2001$ or 5.4% of the reference set (probability 0.054 if the null hypothesis is true). This just fails to reach significance at the 5% level. When we ran the macro again, we had 112 values at least as small as ours, giving a probability of 0.056. The **statistical conclusion** could be reported as follows.

> In a randomization test of the prediction that using a pager would increase the frequency with which our participant would do prescribed exercises, 5.4% of a random sample of 2000 rearrangement statistics were at least as small as our

```
Run MATRIX procedure:

RSS
     1.777777778

count of RSS as least as small
     108

probability
     10 ** -2   X
      5.447276362


------ END MATRIX -----
```

Figure 5.4 *SPSS Output 5.4.* Result from a single-case randomized blocks design.

experimental value. This does not quite reach the 5% significance level, so we do not reject the null hypothesis that the pager makes no difference. Our experiment has not provided evidence significant at the 5% level that using the pager increases the frequency of doing the exercises for this participant.

Notice that in a case like this, where our test statistic is quite close to significance at the 5% level, it would be possible for another run to produce a result with a probability just below 5%. If we are using a random sample from the reference set to estimate the position in the reference set of our actual test statistic, as in all our macros, then a result that only just reaches significance should be reported with a cautionary note or else with the results from several runs. This is discussed fully at the start of Chapter 7.

To use the macro with your own data, just edit the data file but keep the variable names the same.

Analogs of ANOVA: a small-n repeated measures design

This design uses the *randomizedblocks* macro, so open the syntax file *randomizedblocks.sps*. The data for our example are in the file *repeatedmeasures. sav*. Open this, and run the macro in the usual way. In a few seconds, the results appear in the output window as shown in Figure 5.4 *SPSS Output 5.4*. However, for this example we have the actual RSS appearing as 1.33. This is the same as the RSS you would get from a two-way ANOVA with the participants as blocks. On our example run, we found only 13 at least as small as ours in the 2000 sample rearrangements, so our test statistic is in the smallest 14/2001 or 0.7% (probability 0.007 if the null hypothesis is true). The **statistical conclusion** could be reported as follows.

> A randomization test of the null hypothesis that that pager prompts do not alter the number of times patients do their exercises gave 0.7% of a random sample of 2000 rearrangement statistics at least as small as our experimental value. This is significant at the 5% level, so we reject the null hypothesis and conclude that our experiment supports the alternative hypothesis that using the pager affects the number of times patients do their exercises. The means for the three conditions are 0.5, 1.5, and 3.5, suggesting that it may be worth using the double prompt.

Analogs of ANOVA: a single-case randomized blocks design with two conditions

The macro for this design is *randomizedblockstwoconditions.sps*, and the data for this example are *randomizedblockstwoconditions.sav*. Open both the files, and run the macro in the usual way. In a few seconds, the results appear in the output window, as shown in Figure 5.5 *SPSS Output 5.5*.

Our test statistic is 1.6 (drug A mean is 4.6, and drug B mean is 3.0). In our example run, we had 72 rearrangement values at least as large, so our value is in the largest 73/2001 or 4% of the reference set (probability 0.04 if the null hypothesis is true). The **statistical conclusion** could be reported as follows.

```
Run MATRIX procedure:

test statistic
   1.600000000

count of arrangement statistics at least as large
   72

one tail probability
   10 ** -2   X
   3.648175912

count of arrangement statistics at least as large in abs value as abs(test)
   137

two tail probability
   10 ** -2   X
   6.896551724

------ END MATRIX -----
```

Figure 5.5 *SPSS Output 5.5*. Result from a single-case randomized blocks design with two conditions.

In a randomization test of the prediction that drug A will give longer relief from pain than drug B, 4% of a random sample of 2000 rearrangement statistics were at least as large as our experimental value. This result is significant at the 5% level using a one-tailed test: Our data support the view that drug A gives longer relief than drug B.

If we want to use a two-tailed test for an alternative hypothesis that says the drugs differ but without predicting the direction, we ignore the sign of our test statistic and of those calculated from the rearrangements. In this example, we had 137 at least as large as ours, ignoring the signs. So the two-tailed test does not give a significant result (138/2001 is 6.9%).

To run the macro with your own data, just replace our example data with yours, but keep the variable names.

Analogs of ANOVA: a small-n repeated measures design with replicates

The macro for the small-*n* repeated measures design with replicates is *smallgrouprepeatedwithreps.sps,* and the example data file is *smallgroup-repeatedwithreps.sav.* Run the macro in the usual way to obtain the output as shown in Figure 5.6 *SPSS Output 5.6.*

First is the test statistic calculated from the actual data, 1.33 (the condition 2 mean is 4.83, and the condition 1 means is 3.50). Then we have the

```
Run MATRIX procedure:

test statistic
   1.333333333

count of arrangement statistics at least as large
   84

one tail probability
   10 ** -2   X
   4.247876062

count of arrangement statistics at least as large in abs value as abs(test)
   185

two tail probability
   10 ** -2   X
   9.295352324

------ END MATRIX -----
```

Figure 5.6 *SPSS Output 5.6.* Result from a small-*n* repeated-measures design with replicates.

count of reference set values at least as large as our actual test statistic, followed by the one-tailed probability.

A one-tailed test is appropriate here because if there is any difference in perceived depth, the greater perceived depth would be expected for the perspective cue (P). Our result is just significant at the 5% level. However, we should warn you that when we ran this macro again, we obtained a count of 104 values from the reference set at least as large as the actual test statistic, giving a probability slightly above 5%. A random sample of 2000 values gives a good estimate of where our test statistic falls in the reference set, but if your test statistic is rather close to the 5% boundary, you need to be cautious in what you claim. There is further discussion of this at the start of Chapter 7. The **statistical conclusion** could be reported as follows.

> In a randomization test (one-tailed) of the prediction that the perspective cue would give greater depth perception than the texture cue, 4.2% of a random sample of 2000 rearrangement statistics were at least as large as our experimental value. Because this is a little close to the 5% boundary, we took three more random samples of 2000 rearrangement statistics, and found 4.7%, 5.3%, and 4.6% at least as large as our experimental value. So our experiment gives rather weak support to the view that our volunteers perceive greater depth when the pictorial cue is perspective rather than texture gradient.

After the one-tailed results, we have the count of reference set values at least as large in absolute value as the absolute value for the actual test statistic, and the two-tailed probability, not needed in this case.

Analogs of ANOVA: a two-way factorial single-case design

To analyze our example of a two-way factorial single-case design, open the data file *factorialsinglecase.sav* and the syntax file *factorial.sps*, and run the macro exactly as before.

The macro is in two parts, because the levels of each factor have to be correctly ordered in the datasheet outside the matrix language. So the first part of the macro runs and the results for factor 1 appear in the Output window as shown in Figure 5.7 *SPSS Output 5.7(a)*. Then the second part of the macro runs and the results for factor 2 appear as in Figure 5.8 *SPSS Output 5.7(b)*. In each case, the one-tail results are given first, assuming a directional alternative hypothesis predicting a higher mean for level 2 of the factor.

First look at the factor 1 results. We see that the difference between the condition means is 3.875 (the TV allowed mean is 6.250, and the TV banned mean is 2.375). The one-tailed test results are given first, and because we had a directional alternative hypothesis (that banning TV would reduce disturbance), it is the one-tailed result that we use. In our first run, we found that seven rearrangements gave a difference at least as large, so 8/2001 or 0.4% of the reference set is at least as large (probability 0.004). The two-tailed test follows, but we ignore it as for this example the one-tailed test is appropriate.

Now look at the factor 2 results. The actual test statistic was 0.875 (mean for junk food allowed is 4.750 and junk food banned is 3.875). Once again, we use the one-tailed test results because our alternative hypothesis was that banning junk food would reduce disturbance. The one-tailed

```
Run MATRIX procedure:

factor 1 test statistic
   3.875000000

count of arrangement statistics at least as large
   7

 factor 1 one tail probability
   10 ** -3   X
    3.998001000

count of arrangement statistics at least as large in abs value as abs(test)
   10

 factor 1 two tail probability
   10 ** -3   X
    5.497251374

------ END MATRIX -----
```

Figure 5.7 SPSS *Output 5.7(a).* Factor 1 result from a two-way factorial single-case design.

```
Run MATRIX procedure:

factor 2 test statistic
   .8750000000

count of arrangement statistics at least as large
   474

 factor 2 one tail probability
   .2373813093

count of arrangement statistics at least as large in abs value as abs(test)
   939

 factor 2 two tail probability
   .4697651174

------ END MATRIX -----
```

Figure 5.8 SPSS *Output 5.7(b).* Factor 2 result from a two-way factorial single-case design.

results are given first, and in our example run there were 474 arrangements with a test statistic at least as large as ours, so 475/2001 or 24% of the reference set is at least as large. Once again, we can ignore the two-tailed results. The **statistical conclusions** could be reported as follows.

> Randomization tests of the main effects in a 2*2 factorial experiment on a single attention deficit-hyperactivity disorder (ADHD) sufferer were carried out. We use one-tailed tests for both main effects because we predict that banning TV in the bedroom and banning junk food will both reduce night disturbance. In a test of the main effect of banning TV in the bedroom, 0.4% of a random sample of 2000 rearrangement statistics was at least as large as our experimental value. This is much less than 5%, so our experiment provides evidence that banning TV reduced the number of night disturbances. The test of the main effect of banning junk food gave 24% of the random sample of 2000 rearrangement statistics at least as large. This is well above 5%, so we do not have evidence that banning junk food reduces the number of night disturbances.

Analogs of ANOVA: a two-way factorial small-n design

To analyze our example of a two-way factorial small-n design, open the data file *factorialsmallgroup.sav* and the syntax file *factorial.sps*, and run the macro exactly as before. The analysis is just the same as for the single case, and the results appear in two parts in just the same way as in Figures 5.7 and 5.8 (SPSS Output 5.7 (a) and (b)).

If you look at the factor 1 results for this example, you find that the difference between the condition means is 2.75 (the passive play mean is 5.25, and the active play mean is 2.50). Our alternative hypothesis was that active play would reduce problem behavior, so we use the one-tailed test results, which are given first. In our example run, we found seven rearrangements gave a difference at least as large, so 8/2001 or 0.4% of the reference set is at least as large (probability 0.004). We ignore the two-tailed test for factor 1 because the one-tailed test was appropriate.

Now look at the factor 2 results. This time ignore the one-tailed test because we had no directional alternative for factor 2 (playing alone or in a group). For the two-tailed test, the signs are ignored for the actual test statistic and for those in the reference set. The actual test statistic was 0.75 (means were 3.50 for alone and 4.25 for in a group). Our example run gave 921 arrangements with a test statistic at least as large as ours ignoring the signs. We have 922/2001 = 46%, well above 5%, at least as large as ours in the reference set. The **statistical conclusions** could be reported as follows.

> Randomization tests of the main effects in a 2*2 factorial experiment on 16 learning-disabled children were carried out. We used a one-tailed test for the main effect of active or passive play because we predict that active play will reduce problem behavior. We found 0.4% of a random sample of 2000 rearrangement statistics was at least as large as our experimental value. This is much less than 5%,

so our experiment provides evidence that active play reduced problem behavior. We used a two-tailed test for the main effect of playing alone or in a group because if there was a difference, we could not predict its direction. We found 46% of the random sample of 2000 rearrangement statistics at least as large in absolute value as the absolute value of our experimental value. This is well above 5%, so we do not have evidence that playing alone or in a group affects problem behavior.

Phase designs: a single-case AB design

The macro for the single-case AB design is *singlecaseAB.sps*, and the example data file is *singlecaseAB.sav*. Run the macro as usual, and in a few seconds the results appear as shown in Figure 5.9 *SPSS Output 5.8*. First is the test statistic, 11.0 for our example (the intervention mean is 35.0, and the baseline mean is 24.0). Next is the count of rearrangement statistics at least as large, 71 in our example run. This means our test statistic is in the highest 72/2001 or 3.6% of the reference set (probability 0.04 using a one-tailed test). Recall that we predicted that pain distress scores would be reduced by the intervention, and in order to use the macro we had to transform the data by subtracting all the scores from a value greater than all of them (we chose to subtract from 50). The **statistical conclusion** could be reported as follows.

A randomization test (one-tailed) of the prediction that mindfulness training would reduce distress scores for a single chronic pain sufferer gave 3.6% of a random sample of 2000 rearrangement statistics at least as large as our experimental value. We conclude that our experiment does provide evidence that mindfulness training reduced distress scores for our patient.

```
Run MATRIX procedure:

test statistic
    11.03571429

count of arrangement statistics at least as large
    71

one tail probability
    10 ** -2    X
    3.598200900

count of arrangement statistics at least as large in abs value as abs(test)
    71

two tail probability
    10 ** -2    X
    3.598200900

------ END MATRIX -----
```

Figure 5.9 *SPSS Output 5.8.* Results for a single-case AB design.

```
Run MATRIX procedure:

test statistic
   4.000000000

count of arrangement statistics at least as large
   100

one tail probability
   10 ** -2   X
    5.04747 62 62

count of arrangement statistics at least as large in abs value as abs(test)
   100

two tail probability
   10 ** -2   X
    5.04747 62 62

------ END MATRIX -----
```

Figure 5.10 *SPSS Output 5.9*. Results for a single-case ABA design.

We can ignore the two-tailed test results because a directional alternative was appropriate in this example.

Phase designs: a single-case ABA design

The macro for the single-case ABA design is *singlecaseABA.sps*, and the example data file is *singlecaseABA.sav*. Run the macro as usual, and in a few seconds the results appear as shown in Figure 5.10 *SPSS Output 5.9*. First is the test statistic, 4.00 for our example (the intervention mean is 7.33, and the mean for the baseline and withdrawal observations is 3.33). Next is the count of rearrangement statistics at least as large, 100 in our example run. This means our test statistic is in the highest 101/2001, or 5.0% of the reference set (probability 0.05 using a one-tailed test). Our result is on the boundary for significance at the 5% level, and with a result like this from 2000 sampled rearrangement statistics, we might easily find another macro run gives a value that just reaches or just fails to reach significance at the 5% level. This is discussed further at the start of Chapter 7. The **statistical conclusion** could be reported as follows.

A randomization test (one-tailed) of the prediction that providing a list would increase the number of subtasks completed for a successful breakfast for a single head injury patient gave 5.0% of a random sample of 2000 rearrangement statistics at least as large as our experimental value. Our result is on the boundary for significance at the 5% level, so as we used a random sample of 2000 rearrangement statistics, we took three more samples of 2000 rearrangement statistics and found 5.1%, 5.4%, and 5.0% at least as large as our experimental value. Our study provides rather weak support for the view that the checklist increases the number of subtasks completed.

We ignore the two-tailed test results because we had a directional alternative hypothesis.

Phase designs: a multiple baseline AB design

The macro for the multiple baseline AB design is *multiplebaselineAB.sps*, and the example data file is *multiplebaselineAB.sav*. Run the macro in the usual way, and in a few seconds the results appear as shown in Figure 5.11 *SPSS Output 5.10*. For our first measure, competence score, the intervention and baseline means are 5.30 and 4.00 respectively, giving a difference of 1.30. For our second measure, interest score, the means are 7.75 and 3.86, giving a difference of 3.89. Adding the differences, we get our test statistic, 5.19, shown at the start of the output. Then we have the count of reference set values at least as large as this, 23 in our example run. So our value is in the top 24/2001 or 1.2% of the reference set, giving a probability for the one-tailed test of 0.01.

When we find a significant result from a test on the multiple baseline AB design, it means that at least one of the participants or measures shows a significant change. It does not imply a significant change for all participants or measures. The **statistical conclusion** for this example could be reported as follows.

```
Run MATRIX procedure:

test statistic
    5.192857143

count of arrangement statistics at least as large
   23

one tail probability
  10 ** -2    X
   1.199400300

count of arrangement statistics at least as large in abs value as abs(test)
   23

two tail probability
  10 ** -2    X
   1.199400300

------ END MATRIX -----
```

Figure 5.11 *SPSS Output 5.10*. Results for a multiple baseline AB design.

A randomization test (one-tailed) was used to test the prediction that training in the use of turn-around questions and feedback remarks would make a communication aid user appear more competent and more interested, respectively. We found 1.2% of a random sample of 2000 rearrangement statistics was at least as large as our experimental value. This is significant at the 5% level. However, our test statistic combines results from the two kinds of training, so we can say only that at least one of the measures (competence score and interest score) was increased by the intervention directed at it. Looking at the means, we see that although both scores increased after intervention, the increase in the interest score was about three times the increase in the competence score.

We can ignore the two-tailed test because we used directional alternative hypotheses. To use the macro with other data, keep the variable names and replace the data with your own or any other suitable example.

Phase designs: a multiple baseline ABA design

The macro for the multiple baseline ABA design is *multiplebaselineABA.sps*, and the example data file is *multiplebaselineABA.sav*. Run the macro in the usual way, and in a few seconds the results appear as shown in Figure 5.12 *SPSS Output 5.11*. For our first participant, the intervention and baseline–withdrawal means are 9.00 and 2.00, respectively, giving a difference of 7.00. For our second participant, the means are 8.75 and 1.50, giving a difference of 7.25; and for the third participant, the means are 8.67 and 3.00 with a difference of 5.67. Adding the differences we get our test statistic, 19.92, shown at the start of the output. Then we have the count of reference set values at least

```
Run MATRIX procedure:

test statistic
   19.91666667

count of arrangement statistics at least as large
   9

one tail probability
   10 ** -3   X
   4.997501249

count of arrangement statistics at least as large in abs value as abs(test)
   9

two tail probability
   10 ** -3   X
   4.997501249

------ END MATRIX -----
```

Figure 5.12 *SPSS Output 5.11.* Results for a multiple baseline ABA design.

as large as this, 9 in our example run. So our value is in the top 10/2001 or 0.5% of the reference set, giving a probability for the one-tailed test of 0.005.

If we obtain a significant result for the multiple baseline ABA design, we can only claim that at least one participant (or measure) has shown a significant increase in the intervention phase. However, in this example, when we look at the means for the three participants we can see that all three showed some benefit. The **statistical conclusion** for this example could be reported as follows.

> A randomization test (one-tailed) was used to test the prediction that providing a list would increase the number of subtasks successfully completed by three head injury patients. We found 0.5% of a random sample of 2000 rearrangement statistics was at least as large as our experimental value. This is significant at the 5% level, but because our test statistic combines results from the three participants, it tells us only that at least one of our head injury patients achieved a significant increase in breakfast score while using the checklist. However, when we look at the means for the three participants, it appears that all benefited.

Our alternative hypothesis predicted that the checklist would increase scores, so we can ignore the two-tailed results. To use the macro with other data, keep the variable names and replace the data with your own or any other suitable example.

A design to test order effects

The macro for the design to test order effects is *ordereffects.sps*, and the data file for our example is *ordereffects.sav*. Running the macro in the usual way produces output as shown in Figure 5.13 *SPSS Output 5.12*. The test

```
Run MATRIX procedure:

sum of products
   53.75000000

count of arrangement sums of products at least as large
   35

probability
   10 ** -2   X
   1.799100450

------ END MATRIX -----
```

Figure 5.13 SPSS Output 5.12. Results for a design to test order effects.

statistic, 1.63*1 + 1.63*2 + 2.73*3 + 4.33*4 + 4.67*5 = 53.75, is followed by the count of values at least as large from the 2000 sample rearrangements of the predicted order, 35 in our example run. So our test statistic is in the top 36/2001 or 1.8% of the reference set. The probability if the null hypothesis that we cannot predict the order is true is 0.018. The **statistical conclusion** for this example could be reported as follows.

> We used a randomization test (one-tailed) to test the prediction that similar pieces of writing would be arranged in the same order as the familiarity of the names attached to them. We found 1.8% of a random sample of rearrangement statistics was at least as large as our experimental value. This is much less than 5%, so our experiment supports the view that the teachers ranked the writing from best to worst according to the attached names, from most familiar to least familiar.

Analyses using the Excel macros

If you have not used Excel macros before, there are some general instructions for running them in Appendix 3. The macro and data are all in the workbook for Excel. They have all been stored as macro-enabled workbooks with the extension *xlsm*. (You may still have to click **Enable macros** when you open the workbooks.) Usually you can run the macros with your own data just by deleting the example data and entering your own. The variable names, which are at the top of the columns in row 1, should always be kept the same. Four macros, *oneway*, *randomizedblocks*, *multiplebaselineAB*, and *multiplebaselineABA*, assign names to sections of columns so that they can be referred to during parts of the calculations. When entering new data into these macros, it is necessary to edit the range of these names. This is easily done in the **Name Manager** window on the **Formulas** tab, and Appendix 3 explains the process.

The Excel macros are much slower than the SPSS versions, as the operations needed are less efficiently performed by Excel. The slowest ones are the multiple baseline AB and ABA designs, and these may take about 20 minutes, depending on the speed of your computer.

Analogs of ANOVA: a single-case one-way design

Excel keeps the data and macros all in the workbook, and you will find that *oneway.xlsm* contains the macro *oneway* and the data for the single-case example. To run the macro, first click the **Developer** tab on the menu bar, then click the **Macros** button. In the dialog box that appears there is only one macro, so just click **Run**. Refer to Appendix 3 if you are not sure about this.

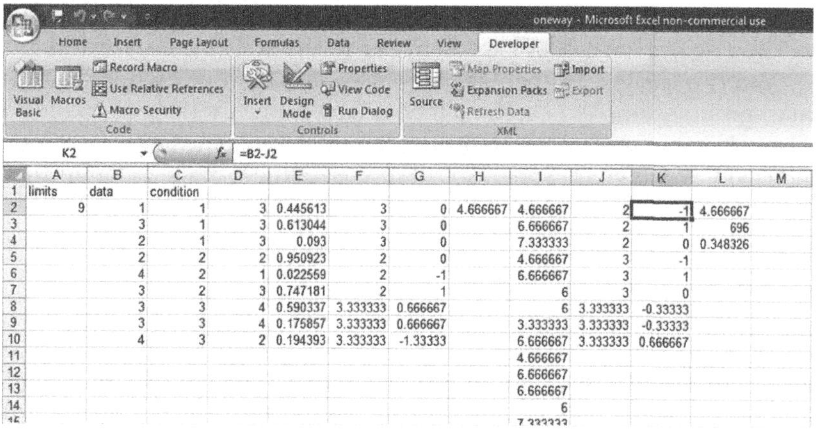

	A	B	C	D	E	F	G	H	I	J	K	L	M
1	limits	data	condition										
2	9	1	1	3	0.445613	3	0	4.666667	4.666667	2	-1	4.666667	
3		3	1	3	0.613044	3	0		6.666667	2	1	696	
4		2	1	3	0.093	3	0		7.333333	2	0	0.348326	
5		2	2	2	0.950923	2	0		4.666667	3	-1		
6		4	2	1	0.022559	2	-1		6.666667	3	1		
7		3	2	3	0.747181	2	1		6	3	0		
8		3	3	4	0.590337	3.333333	0.666667		6	3.333333	-0.33333		
9		3	3	4	0.175857	3.333333	0.666667		3.333333	3.333333	-0.33333		
10		4	3	2	0.194393	3.333333	-1.33333		6.666667	3.333333	0.666667		
11									4.666667				
12									6.666667				
13									6.666667				
14									6				
15									7.333333				

Figure 5.14 *Excel Output 5.1.* Analysis of a single-case one-way design; results in column L.

The results appear in column L as shown in Figure 5.14 *Excel Output 5.1*, but remember that your own runs are unlikely to produce exactly the same counts and probabilities as ours, though the test statistics will be the same. L2 contains the RSS for our actual experiment (4.67 for this example), and L3 contains a count of RSS values from the 2000 sample rearrangements that are at least as small as ours (696 in the example shown). So the probability of a value as extreme as our actual one occurring by chance is 697/2001 or 0.348, which is the value in L4. The **statistical conclusion** could be reported as follows.

> We had three methods to test to see whether we could increase the number of activities in which our patient with Alzheimer's joined. In a randomization test of the null hypothesis that our methods did not affect the number of activities he joined, 35% of a random sample of 2000 rearrangement statistics was at least as small as our experimental value. This does not approach significance at the 5% level, and we conclude that we do not have evidence that our methods affect the number of activities he joined in.

Columns D to K contain the calculations performed by the macro, and you can ignore them.

Notice that because we take a random sample of 2000 rearrangements of the condition labels, if we run the macro again we expect a slightly different number of RSS values at least as small as the actual one. On a rerun, we found 722 values at least as small as the actual one, giving a probability of 0.361.

To run the macro again with the same data, just click the **Macros** button and **Run** again; the columns used by the macro will just be overwritten.

You can easily edit the data to replace it with your own, or with the small-group example data. Keep the variable names at the top of columns A to C, but you will need to edit the range of the names ARRANGE, DATA, and LEVEL as shown in Appendix 3. For each of these names, change the 10 (last row of the example data) to the last row of the new data.

Analogs of ANOVA: a small-n one-way design

Open the Excel workbook *oneway.xlsm*. Excel keeps the data and macros all in the workbook, and you will find that *oneway.xlsm* contains the macro *oneway* and the data for the single case. The data for the small-*n* example appears in Table 4.2. To run the macro with the data for the small-*n* example, first edit the data (using Table 4.2) and the ranges for the names ARRANGE, DATA, and LEVEL so that they end in row 11, as shown in Appendix 3. Once you have the data for the small-*n* example in the datasheet, run the macro as before.

The results appear in column L (see Figure 5.15 *Excel Output 5.2*). L2 contains the RSS for our actual experiment (3.33 for this example), and L3 contains a count of RSS values from the 2000 sample rearrangements that are at least as small as ours (we got 9 on our first run). So the probability of a value as extreme as our actual one occurring by chance is 10/2001

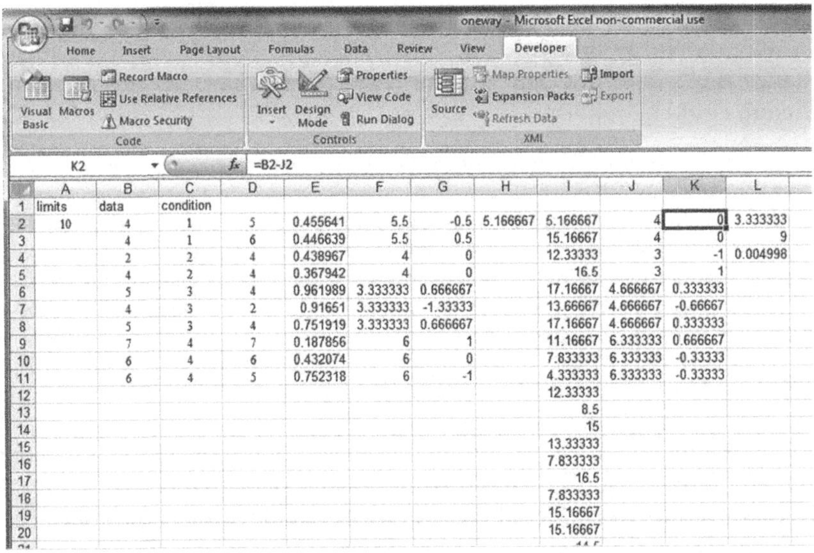

	A	B	C	D	E	F	G	H	I	J	K	L
1	limits	data	condition									
2	10	4	1	5	0.455641	5.5	-0.5	5.166667	5.166667	4	0	3.333333
3		4	1	6	0.446639	5.5	0.5		15.16667	4	0	9
4		2	2	4	0.438967	4	0		12.33333	3	-1	0.004998
5		4	2	4	0.367942	4	0		16.5	3	1	
6		5	3	4	0.961989	3.333333	0.666667		17.16667	4.666667	0.333333	
7		4	3	2	0.91651	3.333333	-1.33333		13.66667	4.666667	-0.66667	
8		5	3	4	0.751919	3.333333	0.666667		17.16667	4.666667	0.333333	
9		7	4	7	0.187856	6	1		11.16667	6.333333	0.666667	
10		6	4	6	0.432074	6	0		7.833333	6.333333	-0.33333	
11		6	4	5	0.752318	6	-1		4.333333	6.333333	-0.33333	
12									12.33333			
13									8.5			
14									15			
15									13.33333			
16									7.833333			
17									16.5			
18									7.833333			
19									15.16667			
20									15.16667			

Figure 5.15 *Excel Output 5.2*. Analysis of a small-*n* one-way design; results in column L.

or 0.005, which is the value in L4. The **statistical conclusion** could be reported as follows.

In a randomization test of the hypothesis that different communication aids would take different lengths of time to learn to a criterion, only 0.5% of a random sample of 2000 rearrangement statistics was at least as small as our experimental value. This is much less than 5%, so we reject the null hypothesis of no difference among times taken to learn to use the aids. Our experiment supports the alternative hypothesis that the different types of communication aid take different lengths of time to learn.

To use the macro with your own data, replace the example data with your own. Remember to edit the name ranges as shown in Appendix 3, and keep the variable names the same.

Analogs of ANOVA: a small-n one-way design with two conditions

The data and macro for our example are in the Excel workbook *oneway-twoconditions.xlsm*. Run the macro in the usual way (refer to Appendix 3 if you are not sure how). Our run took 2 minutes, and the results are shown in Figure 5.16 *Excel Output 5.3*. The difference between the condition means is 2.05 (the passive play mean is 4.25, and the active play mean is 2.20), and column I contains this test statistic at the top. Then in I3, we have the number of rearrangements with a value at least as high for a one-tailed test

	A	B	C	D	E	F	G	H	I	J
	limits	data	condition	arrange						
2	9	4	1	4	0.485244	3.25	0.25	0.25	2.05	
3		4	1	6	0.151464	3	1.15	1.15	161	
4		1	1	2	0.187236	0.25	-0.65	0.65	0.08096	
5		2	1	1	0.101364	0.25	-1.1	1.1	2.05	
6		0	1	2	0.936207	4.25	-2.45	2.45	286	
7		4	2	4	0.002739	2.2	1.15	1.15	0.143428	
8		6	2	0	0.123434	2.05	1.15	1.15		
9		2	2	5	0.170021	2.05	-1.55	1.55		
10		5	2	4	0.931369		0.25	0.25		
11							0.25	0.25		
12							0.7	0.7		
13							0.7	0.7		
14							0.25	0.25		

Figure 5.16 Excel Output 5.3. Analysis of a one-way design with just two conditions; results in column I.

(161 for this run). This gives 162/2001 or 8.1% of the reference set at least as large as our value (probability 0.08 in I4). The **statistical conclusion** could be reported as follows.

> In a randomization test of the prediction that active play reduces problem behavior in a subsequent learning activity in children with learning disabilities, 8.1% of the rearrangement statistics was at least as large as our experimental value. This is not less than 5%, so we do not reject the null hypothesis: Our experiment did not provide evidence that active play reduced problem behavior in a subsequent learning activity.

We should ignore the cells I5–I7 because they give the results for a two-tailed test and we have a directional hypothesis, but we will look at the result. Cells I5 and I6 give the actual test statistic for the two-tailed test and the number of rearrangement values at least as large, ignoring the sign. Because our actual test statistic was positive, ignoring the sign leaves it unchanged, and on this run 286 were at least as large, 287/2001 or 14.3%. This is a probability of 0.143, shown in I6.

To run the macro with different data, just delete the example data in A2 to D10 and replace with the new data. Leave the variable names in row 1 unchanged.

Analogs of ANOVA: a single-case randomized blocks design

Open the Excel workbook *randomizedblocks.xlsm*, which contains the macro and also the data for this example. Run the macro in the usual way, and in about 2 minutes the results appear as shown in Figure 5.17 *Excel Output 5.4*. Cell Q2 contains the actual test statistic (the RSS) from our experiment, 1.78. In Q3 is the number at least as small as ours from the 2000 rearrangements (109 in this run). This means our value was in the smallest 110/2001 or 5.5%, probability 0.055 if the null hypothesis is true. The **statistical conclusion** could be reported as follows.

> In a randomization test of the prediction that using a pager would increase the frequency with which our participant would do prescribed exercises, 5.5% of a random sample of 2000 rearrangement statistics was at least as small as our experimental value. This does not quite reach the 5% significance level, so we do not reject the null hypothesis that the pager makes no difference. Our experiment has not provided evidence significant at the 5% level that using the pager increases the frequency of doing the exercises for this participant.

Notice that in a case like this, where our test statistic is quite close to significance at the 5% level, it would be possible for another run to produce a result with a probability just below 5%. If we are using a random sample from the reference set to estimate the position in the reference set of our

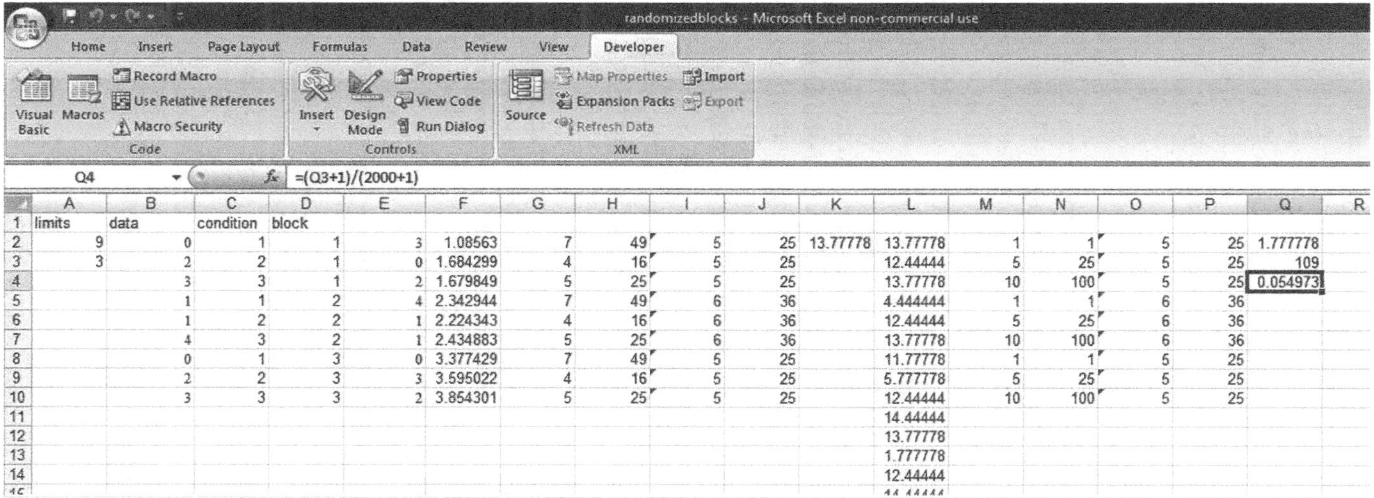

Figure 5.17 Excel Output 5.4. Analysis of a single-case randomized blocks design; results in column Q.

actual test statistic, as in all our macros, then a result that only just reaches significance should be reported with a cautionary note or else with the results from several runs. This is discussed fully at the start of Chapter 7.

To use the macro with your own data, delete the example data in A2 to D10 and replace with the new data. Then edit the name ranges for the names BLOCK, CONDITION, DATA, and PERM, as shown in Appendix 3.

Analogs of ANOVA: a small-n repeated measures design

The macro is in the workbook *randomizedblocks.xlsm*, but the data in the workbook are those for the previous example. To run the macro with the data for the small-*n* example, edit the datasheet, replacing the data in A2 to D10 with the data from Table 4.5. In this case, it is also necessary to edit the ranges of the names BLOCK, CONDITION, DATA, and PERM as shown in Appendix 3. The data for this example occupy rows 2 to 13, so when you finish editing the name ranges, they will all end with the number 13.

The macro takes about 2 minutes to run, and the output appears just as in Figure 5.17 *Excel Output 5.4*, with column Q holding the RSS from our actual experiment, then the count of rearrangements that gave a value at least as small as ours, then the probability of a value this small if the null hypothesis is true. The actual RSS is 1.33, and on our example run we had 19 values at least as low from our sample of 2000 rearrangements. So our value is in the smallest 20/2001 or 1% of the reference set (probability 0.010 if the null hypothesis is true). The **statistical conclusion** could be reported as follows.

> A randomization test of the null hypothesis that that pager prompts do not alter the number of times patients do their exercises gave 1.0% of a random sample of 2000 rearrangement statistics at least as small as our experimental value. This is significant at the 5% level, so we reject the null hypothesis and conclude that our experiment supports the alternative hypothesis that using the pager affects the number of times patients do their exercises. The means for the three conditions are 0.5, 1.5, and 3.5, suggesting that it may be worth using the double prompt.

To run this macro with your own data, delete the data in cells A2 to D13 and enter your own. Keep the variable names the same, but edit the name ranges as shown in Appendix 3 so that the 13s are replaced by the number of your last row of data.

Analogs of ANOVA: a single-case randomized blocks design with two conditions

The macro and example data for this design are in *randomizedblockstwo-conditions.xlsm*. Open the workbook and run the macro in the usual way.

In about 2 minutes, the results appear in the output window as shown in Figure 5.18 *Excel Output 5.5*.

Our test statistic is 1.6 (drug A mean is 4.6, and drug B mean is 3.0), and it appears at the top of column M. In cell M3 is the number of rearrangement values at least as large as ours, 67 in our example run. So our value is in the largest 68/2001 or 3.4% of the reference set (probability 0.034 if the null hypothesis is true, shown in M4). The **statistical conclusion** could be reported as follows.

> In a randomization test of the prediction that drug A will give longer relief from pain than drug B, 3.4% of a random sample of 2000 rearrangement statistics was at least as large as our experimental value. This result is significant at the 5% level using a one-tailed test: Our data support the view that drug A gives longer relief than drug B.

If we want to use a two-tailed test for an alternative hypothesis that says the drugs differ but without predicting the direction, we ignore the sign of our test statistic and of those calculated from the rearrangements. In this example, we had 123 at least as large as ours ignoring the signs (shown in M5). So the two-tailed test does not give a significant result (124/2001 is 6.2%). The two-tailed probability (0.062) is shown in M6.

To run the macro with your own data, just delete the data in cells A2 to D11 and enter your own, but keep the variable names the same.

Analogs of ANOVA: a small-n repeated-measures design with replicates

The macro and our example data for the small-*n* repeated-measures design with replicates is in the Excel workbook *smallgrouprepeatedwithreps.xlsm*. Run the macro in the usual way to get the output as shown in Figure 5.19 *Excel Output 5.6*, with the results in column M.

First is the test statistic calculated from the actual data, 1.33 (the condition 2 mean is 4.83 and the condition 1 mean is 3.50). Then in M3 we have the count of reference set values at least as large as our actual test statistic, followed by the one-tailed probability in M4 (0.048 in our example run). In M5 we have the absolute value of the actual test statistic followed in M6 by the count of absolute values from the reference set for the two-tailed test that are at least as large. Finally in M7 we have the two-tailed probability.

A one-tailed test is appropriate here because if there is any difference in perceived depth we expect the greater depth to be perceived when the pictorial cue is perspective rather than texture gradient. Our result is just significant at the 5% level. A random sample of 2000 values gives a good estimate of where our test statistic falls in the reference set, but if your test

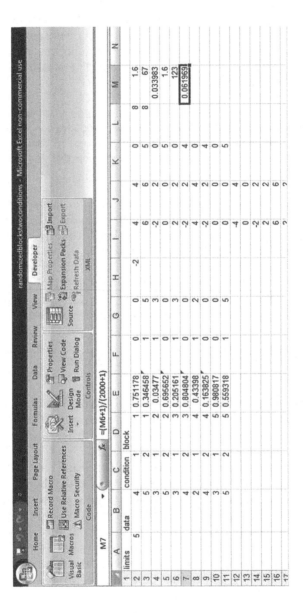

Figure 5.18 Excel Output 5.5. Analysis of a single-case randomized blocks design with two conditions; results in column M.

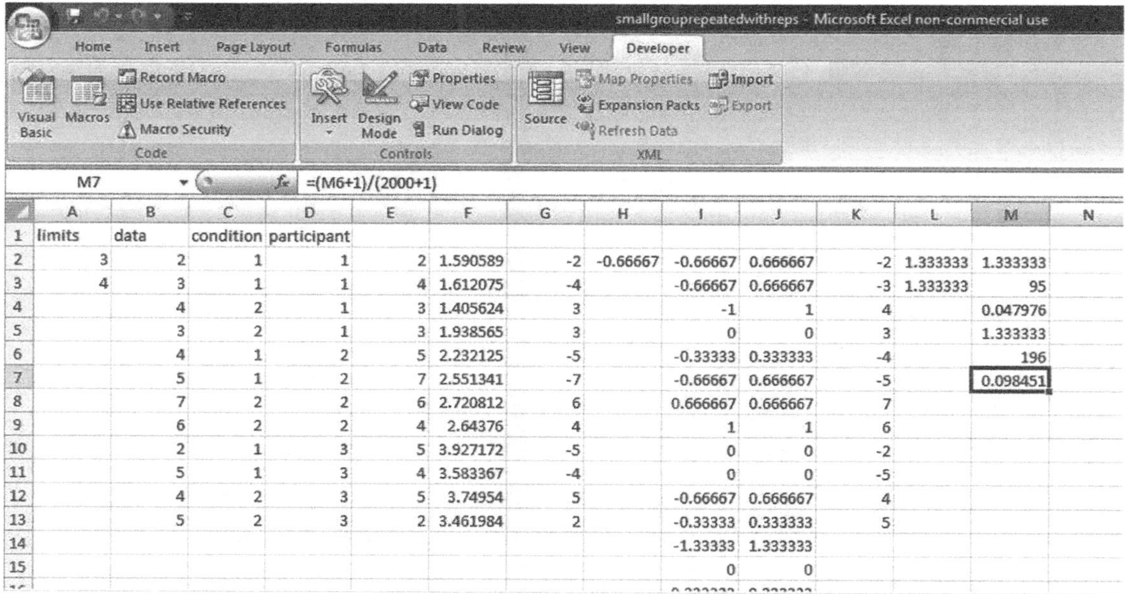

Figure 5.19 *Excel Output 5.6.* Analysis of a small-*n* repeated measures design with replicates; results in column M.

Title bar: smallgouprepeatedwithreps - Microsoft Excel non-commercial use

Ribbon tabs: Home | Insert | Page Layout | Formulas | Data | Review | View | Developer

Code group: Visual Basic, Macros, Record Macro, Use Relative References, Macro Security
Controls group: Insert, Design Mode, Properties, View Code, Run Dialog
XML group: Map Properties, Expansion Packs, Refresh Data, Source, Import, Export

Cell: M7 Formula: =(M6+1)/(2000+1)

	A	B	C	D	E	F	G	H	I	J	K	L	M
1	limits	data	condition	participant									
2		3	2	1	1	1.590589	-2	-0.66667	-0.66667	0.666667	-2	1.333333	1.333333
3		4	3	1	1	1.612075	-4	-0.66667	-0.66667	0.666667	-3	1.333333	95
4			4	2	1	1.405624	3	-1	1	4	4		0.047976
5			3	2	1	1.938565	3	0	0	3	3		1.333333
6			4	1	2	2.232125	-5	-0.33333	-0.33333	0.333333	-4		196
7			5	1	2	2.551341	-7	-0.66667	-0.66667	0.666667	-5		0.098451
8			7	2	2	2.720812	6	0.666667	0.666667	0.666667	7		
9			6	2	2	2.64376	4	1	1	1	6		
10			2	1	3	3.927172	-5	0	0	0	-2		
11			5	1	3	3.583367	-4	0	0	0	-5		
12			4	2	3	3.74954	5	-0.66667	-0.66667	0.666667	4		
13			5	2	3	3.461984	2	-0.33333	-0.33333	0.333333	5		
14								-1.33333	-1.33333	1.333333			
15								0	0	0			

statistic is rather close to the 5% boundary you need to be cautious in what you claim. There is further discussion of this at the start of Chapter 7. The **statistical conclusion** could be reported as follows.

> In a randomization test (one-tailed) of the prediction that the perspective cue would give greater depth perception than the texture cue, 4.8% of a random sample of 2000 rearrangement statistics was at least as large as our experimental value. Because this is rather close to the 5% boundary, we took three more random samples of 2000 rearrangement statistics, and found 4.4%, 5.2%, and 5.3% at least as large as our experimental value. So our experiment gives rather weak support to the view that our volunteers perceive greater depth when the pictorial cue is perspective rather than texture gradient.

Analogs of ANOVA: a two-way factorial single-case design

The macro for the factorial design is in the Excel workbook *factorial.xlsm*. The data for the single-case example are in sheet 1 of the same workbook. To run the macro with the single-case example data, with sheet 1 as the active datasheet, click the **Developer** tab on the menu bar, then the **Macro** button, and then **Run** in the Macro dialog box. After about 2 minutes, the output appears as shown in Figure 5.20 *Excel Output 5.7*, with the results in column U.

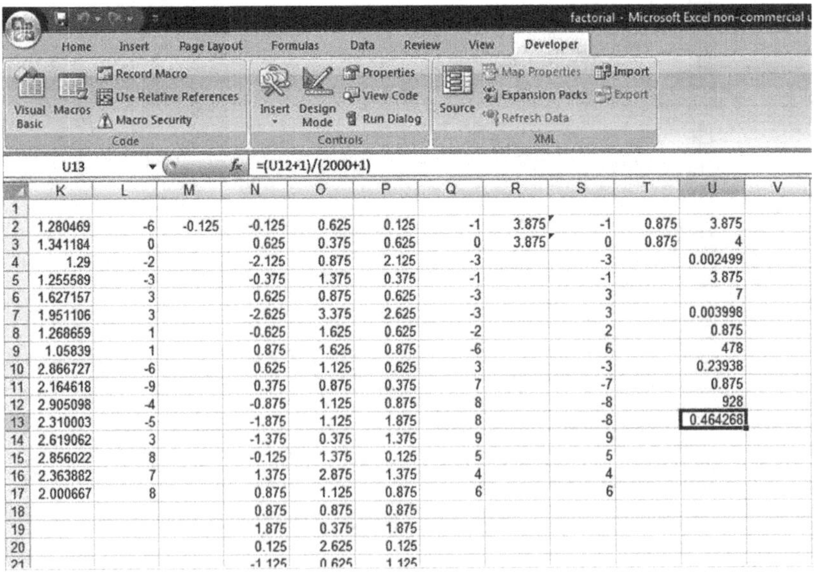

	K	L	M	N	O	P	Q	R	S	T	U	V
1												
2	1.280469	-6	-0.125	-0.125	0.625	0.125	-1	3.875	-1	0.875	3.875	
3	1.341184	0		0.625	0.375	0.625	0	3.875	0	0.875	4	
4	1.29	-2		-2.125	0.875	2.125	-3		-3		0.002499	
5	1.255589	-3		-0.375	1.375	0.375	-1		-1		3.875	
6	1.627157	3		0.625	0.875	0.625	-3		3		7	
7	1.951106	3		-2.625	3.375	2.625	-3		3		0.003998	
8	1.268659	1		-0.625	1.625	0.625	-2		2		0.875	
9	1.05839	1		0.875	1.625	0.875	-6		6		478	
10	2.866727	-6		0.625	1.125	0.625	3		-3		0.23938	
11	2.164618	-9		0.375	0.875	0.375	7		-7		0.875	
12	2.905098	-4		-0.875	1.125	0.875	8		-8		928	
13	2.310003	-5		-1.875	1.125	1.875	8		-8		0.464268	
14	2.619062	3		-1.375	0.375	1.375	9		9			
15	2.856022	8		-0.125	1.375	0.125	5		5			
16	2.363882	7		1.375	2.875	1.375	4		4			
17	2.000667	8		0.875	1.125	0.875	6		6			
18				0.875	0.875	0.875						
19				1.875	0.375	1.875						
20				0.125	2.625	0.125						
21				-1.125	0.625	1.125						

Figure 5.20 *Excel Output 5.7.* Analysis of a single-case factorial design; results in column U.

First we have the test statistic for the main effect of factor 1 in U2. This is 3.875, the difference between the condition means (the TV allowed mean is 6.250, and the TV banned mean is 2.375). In our example run, we found four rearrangements (in U3) with a difference at least as large, so 5/2001 or 0.2% of the reference set is at least as large (probability 0.002, in U4). For the two-tailed test we would find the test statistic in U5, the count of values in the reference set at least as large (ignoring the sign) in U6, and the two-tailed probability in U7. We ignore the two-tailed test for this example because the one-tailed test was appropriate.

The factor 2 results are arranged in exactly the same way in cells U8 to U13. The actual test statistic was 0.875 (mean for junk food allowed is 4.750 and junk food banned is 3.875). For the one-tailed test in our example run there were 478 arrangements with a test statistic at least as large as ours, so 479/2001 or 24% of the reference set is at least as large. Once again, we can ignore the two-tailed results. The **statistical conclusions** could be reported as follows.

> Randomization tests of the main effects in a 2*2 factorial experiment on a single ADHD sufferer were carried out. We used one-tailed tests for both main effects because we predicted that banning TV in the bedroom and banning junk food will both reduce night disturbance. In a test of the main effect of banning TV in the bedroom, 0.2% of a random sample of 2000 rearrangement statistics was at least as large as our experimental value. This is much less than 5%, so our experiment provides evidence that banning TV reduced the number of night disturbances. The test of the main effect of banning junk food gave 24% of the random sample of 2000 rearrangement statistics at least as large. This is well above 5%, so we do not have evidence that banning junk food reduces the number of night disturbances.

To use the macro with your own data, just delete the data in cells A2 to D17 and replace with your own. Remember to use our variable names.

Analogs of ANOVA: a two-way factorial small-n design

The macro for the factorial design is in the Excel workbook *factorial.xlsm*. The data for the small-*n* example are in sheet 2 of the same workbook. To run the macro with the small-*n* example data, sheet 2 must be the active datasheet, then run the macro in the usual way using the **Developer** tab.

The results appear in column U exactly as in the single-case example shown in Figure 5.20 *Excel Output 5.7*, with factor 1 in U2 to U7 (one-tailed followed by two-tailed) and factor 2 in U8 to U13. For this example, the factor 1 test statistic is 2.75 (the passive play mean is 5.25, and the active play mean is 2.50). In our example run, we found eight rearrangement values at least as large as ours for the one-tailed test. So 9/2001 or 0.4% of the reference set is at least as large (probability 0.004). We ignore the two-tailed test for factor 1 because the one-tailed test was appropriate.

For factor 2, we ignore the one-tailed test (in U8 to U10) because we had no directional alternative for factor 2 (alone or in a group). For the two-tailed test, the signs are ignored for the actual test statistic and for those in the reference set. The actual test statistic was 0.75 (mean for alone was 3.50, and for in a group was 4.25). Our example run gave 868 arrangements (in U12) with a test statistic at least as large as ours ignoring the signs. We have 869/2001 = 43%, well above 5%, at least as large as ours in the reference set. The **statistical conclusions** could be reported as follows.

> Randomization tests of the main effects in a 2*2 factorial experiment on 16 learning disabled children were carried out. We used a one-tailed test for the main effect of active or passive play because we predict that active play will reduce problem behavior. We found 0.4% of a random sample of 2000 rearrangement statistics was at least as large as our experimental value. This is much less than 5%, so our experiment provides evidence that active play reduced problem behavior. We used a two-tailed test for the main effect of playing alone or in a group because, if there was a difference we could not predict its direction. We found 43% of the random sample of 2000 rearrangement statistics at least as large in absolute value as the absolute value of our experimental value. This is well above 5%, so we do not have evidence that playing alone or in a group affects problem behavior.

To use the macro with your own data, just delete the values in A2 to D17 and enter your own. Remember to use our variable names.

Phase designs: a single-case AB design

The Excel macro and example data for the single-case AB design are in *singlecaseAB.xlsm*. Run the macro in the usual way to get the results in column O as shown in Figure 5.21 *Excel Output 5.8*. First in O2 is the test statistic for our experiment, 11.0 (the intervention mean is 35.0 and the baseline mean is 24.0). Next is the count of rearrangement statistics at least as large, 76 in our example run. This means our test statistic is in the highest 77/2001 or 3.8% of the reference set (probability 0.038 using a one-tailed test, O4). Recall that we predicted that pain distress scores would be reduced by the intervention, and in order to use the macro we had to transform the data by subtracting all the scores from a value greater than all of them (we chose to subtract from 50). The **statistical conclusion** could be reported as follows.

> A randomization test (one-tailed) of the prediction that mindfulness training would reduce distress scores for a single chronic pain sufferer gave 3.8% of a random sample of 2000 rearrangement statistics at least as large as our experimental value. We conclude that our experiment does provide evidence that mindfulness training reduced distress scores for our patient.

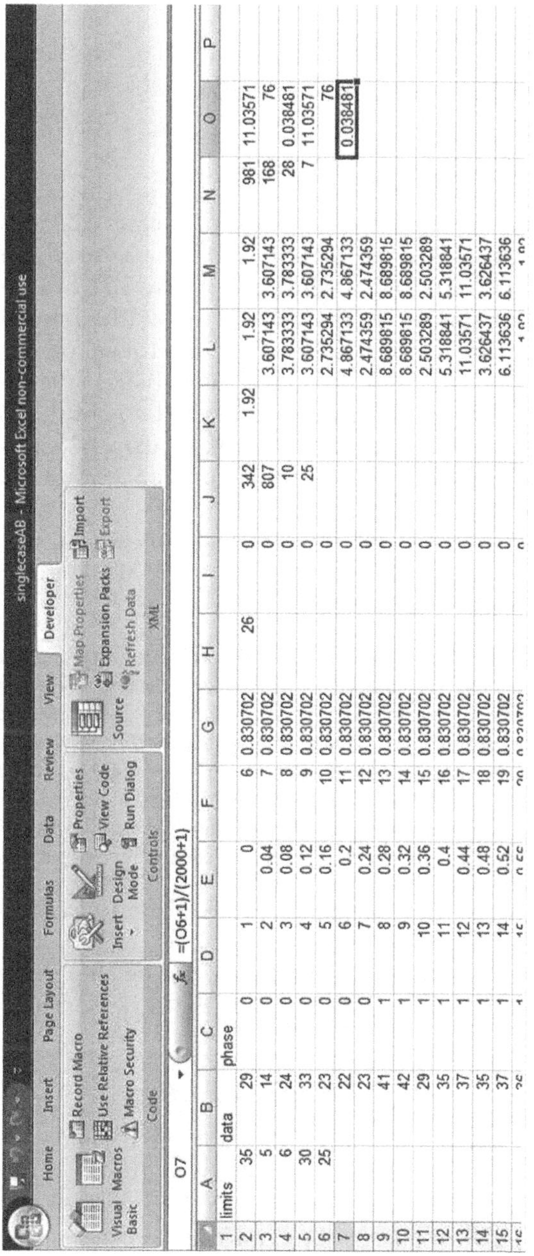

	A	B	C	D	E	F	G	H	I	J	K	L	M	N	O	P
1	limits	data	phase													
2	35	29	0	1	0	6	0.830702	26	0	342	1.92	1.92	1.92	981	11.03571	
3	5	14	0	2	0.04	7	0.830702		0	807		3.607143	3.607143	168	76	
4	6	24	0	3	0.08	8	0.830702		0	10		3.783333	3.783333	28	0.038481	
5	30	33	0	4	0.12	9	0.830702		0	25		3.607143	3.607143	7	11.03571	
6	25	23	0	5	0.16	10	0.830702		0			2.735294	2.735294		76	
7		22	0	6	0.2	11	0.830702		0			4.867133	4.867133		0.038481	
8		23	0	7	0.24	12	0.830702		0			2.474359	2.474359			
9		41	1	8	0.28	13	0.830702		0			8.689815	8.689815			
10		42	1	9	0.32	14	0.830702		0			8.689815	8.689815			
11		29	1	10	0.36	15	0.830702		0			2.503289	2.503289			
12		35	1	11	0.4	16	0.830702		0			5.318841	5.318841			
13		37	1	12	0.44	17	0.830702		0			11.03571	11.03571			
14		35	1	13	0.48	18	0.830702		0			3.626437	3.626437			
15		37	1	14	0.52	19	0.830702		0			6.113636	6.113636			

***Figure 5.21** Excel Output 5.8.* Analysis of a single-case AB design; results in column O.

We ignore the two-tailed test results in O5 to O7 because in this example, we had a directional alternative (pain distress scores decrease after mindfulness training).

To run the macro with your own data, just delete the data in A2 to C36 and replace with your own, but keep the variable names the same.

Phase designs: a single-case ABA design

The macro and example data for the single-case ABA design are in the Excel workbook *singlecaseABA.xlsm*. Run the macro in the usual way to get the results in column R, as shown in Figure 5.22 *Excel Output 5.9*. First in R2 is the test statistic from our study, 4.00 (the intervention mean is 7.33, and the mean for the baseline and withdrawal observations is 3.33). Next in R3 is the count of rearrangement statistics at least as large, 98 in our example run. This means our test statistic is in the highest 99/2001 or 4.9% of the reference set (probability 0.049 using a one-tailed test). Our result is just significant at the 5% level, but with a result as close as this to the 5% boundary from 2000 sampled values we might easily find another run gives a value that just fails to reach significance at the 5% level. This is discussed further at the start of Chapter 7. The **statistical conclusion** could be reported as follows.

> A randomization test (one-tailed) of the prediction that providing a list would increase the number of subtasks completed for a successful breakfast for a single head injury patient gave 4.9% of a random sample of 2000 rearrangement statistics at least as large as our experimental value. As this result is so close to the 5% boundary and we used a random sample of rearrangement statistics, we took three more samples of 2000 rearrangements statistics and found 4.1%, 4.5%, and 5.8% at least as large as our experimental value. Our study gives rather weak support to the view that the checklist increases the number of subtasks completed.

We can ignore the two-tailed results in R5 to R7 because we had a directional alternative hypothesis.

To use the macro with different data, just delete the data in A2 to C16 and replace with the new data, but keep the variable names the same.

Phase designs: a multiple baseline AB design

The example data and macro for the multiple baseline AB design are in *multiplebaselineAB.xlsm*. Running the macro in the usual way produces the results in column S as shown in Figure 5.23 *Excel Output 5.10*. This macro is quite slow and will take about 15 minutes to run.

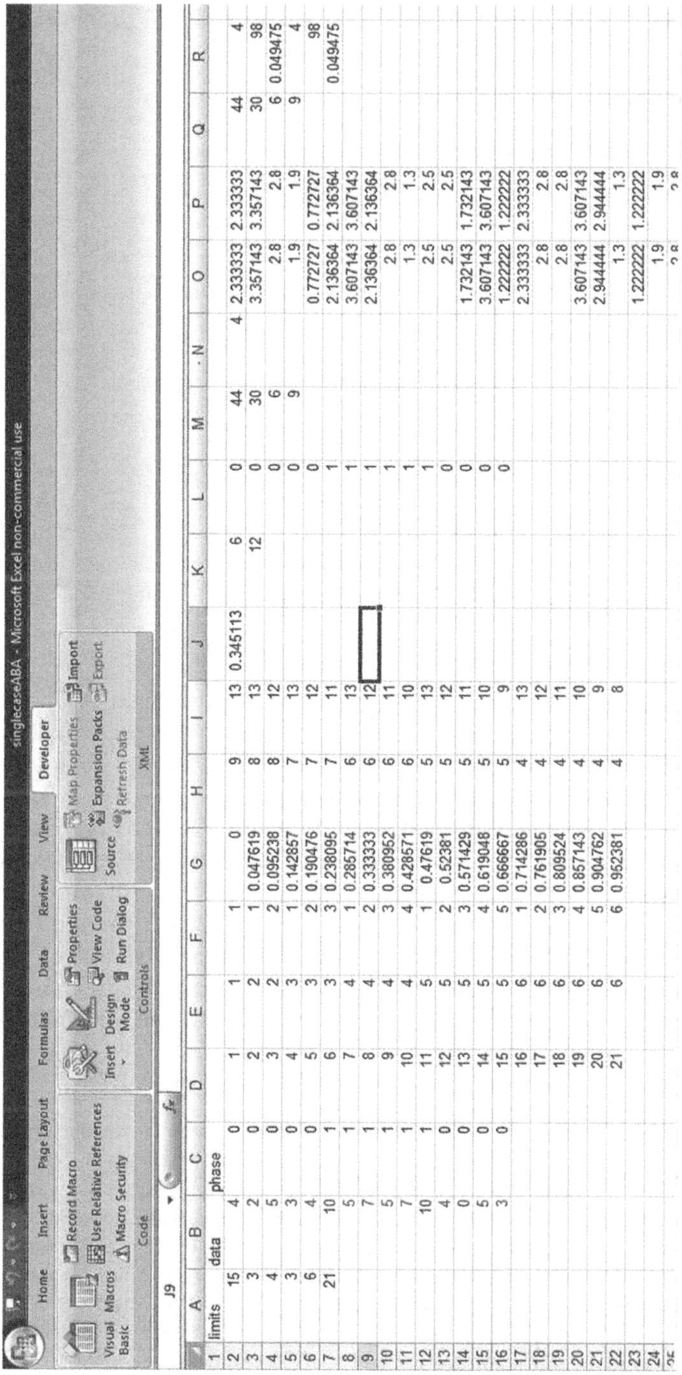

Figure 5.22 Excel Output 5.9. Analysis of a single-case ABA design; results in column R.

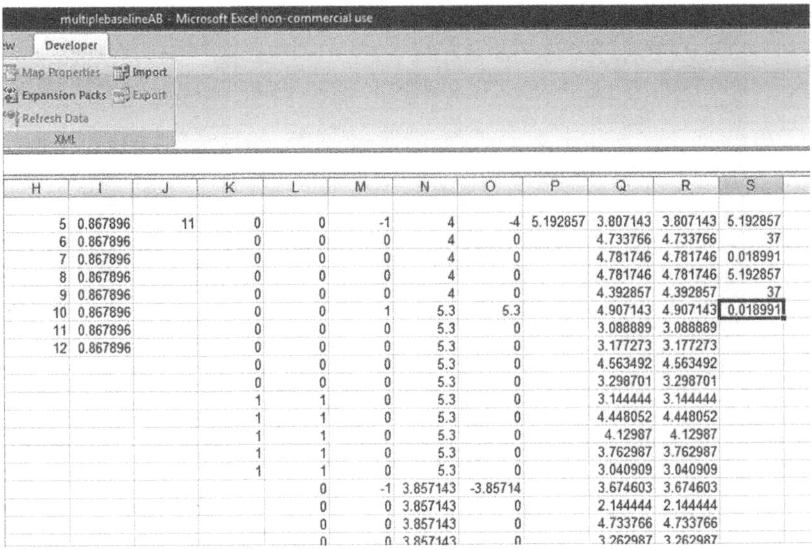

H	I	J	K	L	M	N	O	P	Q	R	S
5	0.867896	11	0	0	-1	4	-4	5.192857	3.807143	3.807143	5.192857
6	0.867896		0	0	0	4	0		4.733766	4.733766	37
7	0.867896		0	0	0	4	0		4.781746	4.781746	0.018991
8	0.867896		0	0	0	4	0		4.781746	4.781746	5.192857
9	0.867896		0	0	0	4	0		4.392857	4.392857	37
10	0.867896		0	0	1	5.3	5.3		4.907143	4.907143	0.018991
11	0.867896		0	0	0	5.3	0		3.088889	3.088889	
12	0.867896		0	0	0	5.3	0		3.177273	3.177273	
			0	0	0	5.3	0		4.563492	4.563492	
			0	0	0	5.3	0		3.298701	3.298701	
			1	1	0	5.3	0		3.144444	3.144444	
			1	1	0	5.3	0		4.448052	4.448052	
			1	1	0	5.3	0		4.12987	4.12987	
			1	1	0	5.3	0		3.762987	3.762987	
			1	1	0	5.3	0		3.040909	3.040909	
				0	-1	3.857143	-3.85714		3.674603	3.674603	
				0	0	3.857143	0		2.144444	2.144444	
				0	0	3.857143	0		4.733766	4.733766	
				0	0	3.857143	0		3.262987	3.262987	

Figure 5.23 *Excel Output 5.10.* Analysis of a multiple baseline AB design; results in column S.

For our first measure, competence score, the intervention and baseline means are 5.30 and 4.00 respectively, giving a difference of 1.30. For our second measure, interest score, the means are 7.75 and 3.86, giving a difference of 3.89. Adding the differences we get our test statistic, 5.19, shown in S2. In S3 is the count of reference set values at least as large as ours, 37 for our example run. This puts our test statistic in the top 38/2001 or 1.9% of the reference set.

When we find a significant result from a test on the multiple baseline AB design, it means that at least one of the participants or measures shows a significant change. It does not imply a significant change for all participants or measures. The **statistical conclusion** for this example could be reported as follows.

> A randomization test (one-tailed) was used to test the prediction that training in the use of turn-around questions and feedback remarks would make a communication aid user appear more competent and more interested, respectively. We found 1.9% of a random sample of 2000 rearrangement statistics was at least as large as our experimental value. This is significant at the 5% level. However, our test statistic combines results from the two kinds of training, so we can say only that at least one of the measures (competence score and interest score) was increased by the intervention directed at it. Looking at the means, we see that although both scores increased after intervention, the increase in the interest score was about three times the increase in the competence score.

We can ignore the two-tailed results in S5 to S7 because our alternative hypotheses were that the interventions would increase scores.

To use the macro with different data, replace the values in A2 to D31 by the new data, keeping the variable names the same. It is also necessary to edit the name ranges as shown in Appendix 3. In this case, the ranges for the names DATA and LEVEL need 31 (the bottom row of example data) replaced by the number of the bottom row of new data.

Phase designs: a multiple baseline ABA design

The example data and macro for the multiple baseline ABA design are in *multiplebaselineABA.xlsm*. Running the macro in the usual way produces the results in column V as shown in Figure 5.24 *Excel Output 5.11*. This macro is quite slow and will take about 20 minutes to run.

For our first participant, the intervention and baseline–withdrawal means are 9.00 and 2.00 respectively, giving a difference of 7.00. For our second participant, the means are 8.75 and 1.50, giving a difference of 7.25, and for the third participant the means are 8.67 and 3.00 with a difference of 5.67. Adding the differences we get our test statistic, 19.92, shown in V2. In V3 is the count of reference set values at least as large as ours, 6 for our example run. This puts our test statistic in the top 7/2001 or 0.3% of the reference set. The one-tailed probability, 0.003, is in V4.

If we obtain a significant result for the multiple baseline ABA design, we can only claim that at least one participant (or measure) has shown a significant increase in the intervention phase. However, in this example, when we look at the means for the three participants we can see that all three showed some benefit. The **statistical conclusion** for this example could be reported as follows.

> A randomization test (one-tailed) was used to test the prediction that providing a list would increase the number of subtasks successfully completed by three head injury patients. We found 0.3% of a random sample of 2000 rearrangement statistics was at least as large as our experimental value. This is significant at the 5% level, but because our test statistic combines results from the three participants, it tells us only that at least one of our head injury patients achieved a significant increase in breakfast score while using the checklist. However, when we look at the means for the three participants, it appears that all benefited.

Because our alternative hypothesis was that the checklist would increase scores, we can ignore the two-tailed results in V5 to V7.

To use the macro with different data, delete the data in A2 to D31 and replace with the new data. Keep the variable names the same but edit name ranges as shown in Appendix 3 for the names DATA and LEVEL used in the macro by replacing 31 (the last row of example data) by the last row of the new data.

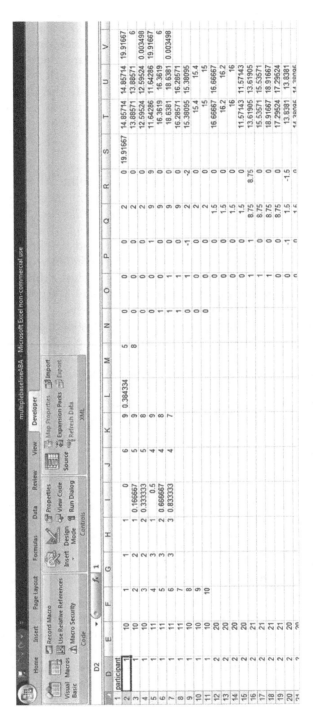

Figure 5.24 Excel Output 5.11. Analysis of a multiple baseline ABA design; results in column V.

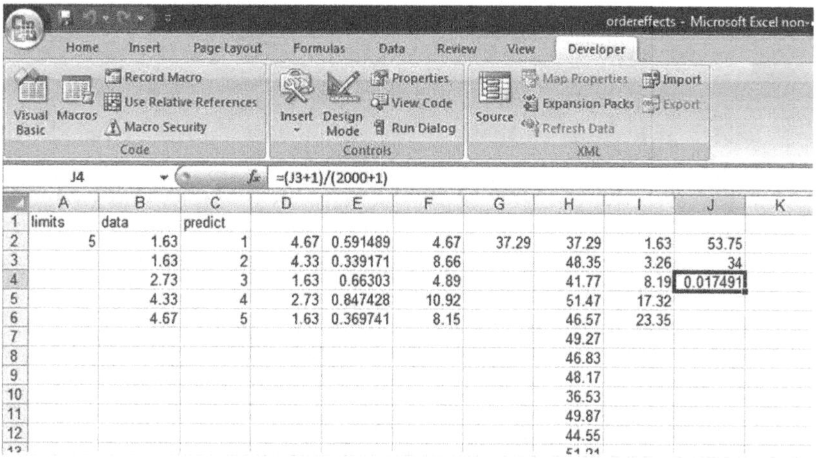

	A	B	C	D	E	F	G	H	I	J	K
1	limits	data	predict								
2	5	1.63	1	4.67	0.591489	4.67	37.29	37.29	1.63	53.75	
3		1.63	2	4.33	0.339171	8.66		48.35	3.26	34	
4		2.73	3	1.63	0.66303	4.89		41.77	8.19	0.017491	
5		4.33	4	2.73	0.847428	10.92		51.47	17.32		
6		4.67	5	1.63	0.369741	8.15		46.57	23.35		
7								49.27			
8								46.83			
9								48.17			
10								36.53			
11								49.87			
12								44.55			

Figure 5.25 *Excel Output 5.12*. Analysis of a design to test order effects; results in column J.

A design to test order effects

The macro and example data for the design to test order effects are in *ordereffects.xlsm*. Running the macro in the usual way produces output as shown in Figure 5.25 *Excel Output 5.12*, with the results in column J. The test statistic, 1.63*1 + 1.63*2 + 2.73*3 + 4.33*4 + 4.67*5 = 53.75, is in J2, followed by the count of values at least as large from the 2000 sample rearrangements of the predicted order, 34 in our example run (J3). So our test statistic is in the top 35/2001 or 1.7% of the reference set. The probability if the null hypothesis that we cannot predict the order is true is 0.017, in J4. The **statistical conclusion** could be reported as follows.

> We used a randomization test (one-tailed) to test the prediction that similar pieces of writing would be arranged in the same order as the familiarity of the names attached to them. We found 1.7% of a random sample of rearrangement statistics at least as large as our experimental value. This is much less than 5%, so our experiment supports the view that the teachers ranked the writing from best to worst according to the attached names, from most familiar to least familiar.

To use the macro with your own data, just delete the data in A2 to C6 and enter any other suitable data in columns A to C but leave the variable names the same.

Exercises

1. If your run, using any of our macros, produces 105 reference set values at least as extreme as the actual test statistic, what do you conclude?

2. When will the test statistic be the same for the one- and two-tailed tests?

3. For users of SPSS, why does output from SPSS macros feature the word MATRIX?

4. For users of Excel, if you get an error using the Excel macro for the multiple baseline AB design with your own data, what might the problem be?

5. For users of Excel, can you suggest why we didn't put the small-*n* example data in sheet 2 for the Excel one-way macro? (*Hint*: Think about the name ranges.)

chapter six

Analyzing the data
Wider considerations

Introduction: the myth of the random sample

Random sampling from a large, well-defined population or universe is a formal requirement for the usual interpretation of all commonly used parametric and nonparametric statistical inferential tests such as the chi-squared test for association, *t* test, and ANOVA. It is also often the justification for a claim of generalizability or external validity. However, usually it is difficult or prohibitively expensive even to define and list the population of interest, a prerequisite of random sampling. As an example of the difficulty of definition, consider the population of "households." Do a landlord and the student lodger doing his or her own shopping and cooking constitute two households or one? What if the landlord provides the student with an evening meal? How many households are there in student flats where they all have their own rooms and share some common areas? And how can the households of interest be listed? Only if we have a list can we take a random sample, and even then it may be difficult. All the full-time students at a university will be on a list and even have a unique registration number, but the numbers will not usually form a continuous series, so random sampling will require the allocation of new numbers. This kind of exercise is usually prohibitively expensive in time, effort, and money, so it is not surprising that samples used in experiments are rarely random samples from any population.

Edgington and Onghena (2007) and Manley (2007), among others, have made the same point for conventional statistical analysis. It is virtually unheard of for experiments with people to meet the random sampling assumption underlying the significance tables that are used to draw inferences about populations. It is difficult to conclude other than that random sampling in human experimental research is little more than a convenient fiction. In reality, generalization almost invariably depends upon replication and nonstatistical reasoning.

In this chapter, we consider how random allocation of conditions to participants or observation occasions, or randomization of an intervention in phase designs, can give us confidence in the internal validity of an experiment. We also discuss how external validity depends on repeating the experiment in different situations, just as when conventional parametric and nonparametric statistics are used. We briefly review the argument that classical parametric tests, as generally used without proper random sampling, are ultimately legitimated by randomization tests.

We show that, even if there is no intention to go beyond graphical analysis of results from a phase design, it is still worth randomizing the intervention point. In the last section, we discuss the use of randomization tests in some situations where randomization is incomplete.

Randomization

In this section, we discuss random assignment of conditions to participants or observation occasions and its effect on internal validity. This effect is independent of whether a randomization test is to be used, or some other statistical test, or visual and graphical analysis only. In fact, randomization is part of good experimental practice, but it also brings with it the advantage that a randomization test can be used.

Randomization tests do not depend on random sampling from a population for their internal validity, as we explained briefly in Chapter 2. All that is required is that conditions are assigned at random to participants or observation occasions, or in the case of phase designs, intervention points are chosen at random from those available. This means that randomization tests are very versatile, in the sense that if a randomization procedure is used in the design of an experiment, then usually an appropriate randomization test can be devised for it. In fact, randomization tests can be carried out for designs (such as phase designs) for which no standard parametric or rank test exists.

The downside to this versatility is that there are numerous ways in which randomization can be introduced into experimental designs, and for each a different randomization test should be specified. It is difficult to generalize the tests, though some general principles can be applied. In Chapters 3 to 5, we demonstrated some of the most common examples of randomization procedures, each with easy-to-use macros to do the appropriate test in SPSS or Excel. In Chapter 8, we will provide some guidance for readers who are interested in writing their own macros or adapting ours to match their own designs. We also provide some information about other software for randomization tests.

In Chapter 3 we briefly mentioned the effect of randomization on internal validity. Phase designs present particular problems in achieving internal validity, and we take up those issues in the later section on phase designs. For now, we discuss randomization and its effect on internal validity for other designs a bit more fully. We also discuss how external validity is achieved, both in the case of randomization tests and where classical statistical methods are used.

The effect on internal validity

The internal validity of an experiment depends on there being no discrete or continuous nuisance variables that exert a biasing (or *confounding*) effect. These variables are *systematic* nuisance variables, and here is an example. A new cancer treatment is to be the subject of a clinical trial, and because the treatment will be arduous for the patients, the doctor in charge admits for the new treatment only those he judges to be sufficiently resolute and optimistic. The others will receive the standard treatment, but these two groups will not be comparable, because patients' mood and attitude may influence the outcome of whatever treatment is given. So the mood and attitude of the patients would be a systematic nuisance variable or confounding effect in this design.

To avoid this problem, we should randomly assign patients to the new or standard treatment, and then their mood and attitude will be a *random* nuisance variable. Although there might be a random effect on the treatment for any particular allocation, these will balance out in the long run. Even if there is no difference in effectiveness between the treatments, it is still possible that by chance those randomly allocated to the new treatment do better just because they happen to have more relevant individual factors such as a more optimistic attitude, but if we use a 5% significance level, then overall we shall reject a true null hypothesis only about 5% of the time.

If we believe that only resolute and optimistic patients can be given the new treatment, then we need to assess each patient for suitability, and those who are suitable for the new treatment are the ones who will enter the trial. Then we randomly assign those in the trial to the new or standard treatment. Any patients not in the trial will receive the standard treatment and will not be included in the comparison of results.

Randomization can turn a potential systematic nuisance variable into a random nuisance variable. If we fail to do this, then a systematic nuisance variable may offer an alternative explanation of any observed effect. In our example where the doctor assigned only resolute and optimistic patients to the new treatment while assigning the less resolute to the standard treatment, it is possible that the most resolute do better than those who are not so positive, regardless of treatment. If our design does not allow for such effects, then statistical tests can do nothing to rescue the internal validity of the study. The only remedy is to build random allocation procedures into the study design at the outset. What random allocation of treatments to participants or observation occasions achieves is that potentially *systematic* nuisance variables (like attitude or mood, in our example) are made into *random* nuisance variables.

When potentially systematic nuisance variables have been converted into random variables by random allocation, they remain a nuisance, but not because they compromise the internal validity of the study. Rather, they are a nuisance because they increase random variability or may interact with a factor. A small but perhaps clinically important effect may not be seen if data from participants are very variable. Of course, if we try to identify a homogeneous group of participants for our study (as the doctor might have done above), then it may not be clear whether the results will apply to other types of patient. We return to this in the "External Validity" section of this chapter.

There is another way in which random variation can obscure any treatment effect. The effects of random variation may happen (by chance) to favor one group or the other. If more patients with a positive attitude happen to be randomly assigned to the new treatment group, resulting in a greater average improvement by that group compared with the old treatment group, their greater improvement might be mistaken for the superior effect of the new treatment. This is where statistical analysis comes in. The statistical analysis, in this case, would tell us how improbable a difference between groups as big as or bigger than that actually obtained would be if only random nuisance variables were responsible. If the probability is less than some agreed criterion (usually 0.05 or 0.01), we will conclude that the difference was unlikely to have been caused by uncontrolled random variables. That leaves us free to infer (provided the experiment is internally valid) that the difference was probably caused by the independent variable (the superiority of the new treatment, in our example).

We cannot emphasize too strongly that the main reason for random assignment of conditions is to secure internal validity, and this is entirely separate from the question of whether to use a randomization test, some other statistical test, or graphical and visual analysis only.

External validity

By *external validity*, we mean the extent to which the results found in our experiment can be applied to patients or others in the world outside our laboratory. In the classical statistical tradition, external validity is ensured by random sampling from the population where we hope to apply the experimental results. The assumption is that we take a random sample from the population of interest, and then whatever we find from the experiment will apply in that population. However, as we pointed out at the start of this chapter, it is almost unknown for experiments involving people to be based on random samples.

In practice, researchers do not invoke the random sampling assumption to claim that their results apply beyond the experimental setting. If potentially useful results are found from an experiment, then the experiment will be repeated in other places with different groups of participants, and if similar results are obtained in different places and with participants whose characteristics vary, we begin to believe in their wide applicability. We also use background knowledge and common sense. If we find a way to increase cooperation among students in our university psychology class, we might expect that the social science students will respond similarly, but we would not expect primary school children to respond in the same way. To find out whether younger students with a wider ability range show similar results, we would need a new experiment. In other words, even when we use classical statistical analysis, external validity is achieved by replication and nonstatistical reasoning, not by random sampling.

We can use randomization tests without assuming anything about how the participants are recruited: All that is needed is that conditions are randomly assigned. But if the participants are not sampled from a well-defined population, how can we generalize the results? We achieve external validity in exactly the same way as is done in practice when using classical statistics: We rely on replication and nonstatistical reasoning. As Edgington and Onghena (2007) said, "The main burden of generalizing from experiments always has been, and must continue to be, carried by nonstatistical rather than statistical logic" (p. 8).

The validity of classical tests

Randomization tests are not a new idea. R. A. Fisher (1935), the great polymath and statistician, described a thought experiment that he called "the lady tasting tea," which is an exact analogy of the ESP experiment described in Chapter 2. Fisher describes an experiment to test a lady's claim that she can tell whether the tea or the milk is poured into the cup first. He proposed presenting eight cups in random order, four each with milk or tea poured first, and explained how to analyze the results using randomization just as we have in the one-way design.

The reason for the late uptake of randomization tests, as we said earlier, is the prodigious amount of computing that is often required. But Fisher believed that other approaches to statistical inference were justified only when randomization tests gave similar results. Edgington and Onghena (2007) gave a brief review of similar views expressed by some of the key figures in 20th-century statistics, including (as well as Fisher), Kempthorne, Winer, Tukey, and the U.S. Statistical Task Force, the latter of which was established to advise on the analysis of weather modification data. Howell (2010) also, in his comprehensive guide to statistics for psychologists, included an introduction to randomization tests. He said, "I believe that in a short time they will overtake what are now the more common nonparametric tests, and may eventually overtake the traditional parametric tests" (p. 660).

Far from regarding classical parametric tests as the gold standard for statistical inference, and randomization tests as a slightly eccentric approach suitable only when we have a single case or small group of participants, it is the randomization tests that provide the gold standard. To summarize, randomization is the key to internal validity, randomization tests do not need the unrealistic assumptions of classical tests (including random sampling), and external validity is achieved by nonstatistical means whether we use randomization or more familiar tests.

Now we consider the special case of phase designs, for which there are no analogous classical tests, and where the importance of randomization to secure internal validity has not always been appreciated.

Phase designs: response guided intervention

When phase designs are used, it is common for the decision when to switch from one phase to another, especially from a baseline phase to a treatment phase, to be based on the pattern of responses in the baseline phase. The widely accepted practice is to continue with baseline observations until the baseline has stabilized, that is, it is reasonably smooth and shows no further evidence of a trend, or at least no trend in the direction predicted for the treatment phase. This is what Morgan and Morgan (2003) called the "steady-state strategy." They summed up current practice:

> Single-participant researchers argue that meaningful effects of an independent variable ought to be noticeable on visual inspection, particularly when the full power of the steady-state strategy is used. Thus visual inspection of dependent measures during independent variable conditions, relative to baseline measures, represents the standard treatment of single-participant data. (p. 644)

Schlosser (2009) quoted the attainment of a steady state as one of the criteria that would indicate the appropriate use of a single-subject experimental design for the identification of empirically supported treatments: "The measurement of baseline data should continue until performance is sufficiently consistent before intervention is introduced to allow prediction of future performance."

It is true that, if baseline responses are highly variable and particularly if they already show a trend similar to that predicted for the treatment phase, it will be difficult to argue that the treatment was effective. It is no solution, however, to resort to response-guided timing of the intervention. In fact, when the timing decision is determined by a rule based on the pattern of baseline responses, any claim to internal validity goes out of the window.

The reason why internal validity cannot be established when the timing of the intervention is response guided is that there is no way of telling what the baseline would have looked like if it had been allowed to continue for a few more observations. We know that it probably would have appeared less stable if we had stopped it a few observations earlier; otherwise, we would have stopped it then. It might also have looked less stable if we had waited for a few more baseline observations before introducing the intervention. After all, we stopped when things seemed to be going particularly well. Perhaps that was just a lucky sequence of trials. One of the difficulties is that intuition is often misleading. We are dealing with probabilities, and in these kinds of experiments we are unlikely to have much idea of the probability of a run of similar responses being followed by a run of increasing or decreasing ones, all of them being nothing more than random variation. In fact, if the responses form an entirely random sequence, then a run of similar values is quite likely to be followed by a run of values that look like a trend up or down.

We have described an alternative way to implement AB designs, in which the total number of available sessions is decided beforehand, along with the minimum number required in the baseline and intervention phases. The intervention point is then chosen at random from those available. For example, if there were to be a total of 15 sessions, with at least 4 sessions in both baseline and treatment phases, the session on which the intervention is introduced is randomly selected from among sessions 5, 6, 7, 8, 9, 10, 11, and 12. If the researcher is unsure how many baseline sessions are required to achieve a reasonable level of stability, a simple modification can be used. All that is necessary is to run *prebaseline* sessions until a stability criterion is reached, *then* begin the baseline sessions followed by the treatment sessions, with the latter commencing at the randomly determined intervention session. This increases the total number of sessions required, but that seems a small price for an internally valid experiment.

If a response-guided procedure is used, it is predictable that the probability of inferring an effect when the null hypothesis is true will increase. This will be true regardless of whether inferences are based on visual or statistical analysis. With regard to visual analysis, Franklin et al. (1996, pp. 139ff.) concluded from a review of studies "evaluating the performance of visual analysis" that the increase in the percentage of false positive results is likely to be substantial. Just *how* substantial will certainly depend on characteristics of the data, such as the extent of serial correlation and learning or practice effects that occur irrespective of the treatment intervention. We demonstrated just how powerful the response guidance bias can be with an illustrative example (Todman & Dugard, 1999), which we will repeat here.

An example of bias when the intervention is response guided

To demonstrate how easy it is to be misled if we don't randomize the intervention point, we simulated some data using an entirely random process in which there was certainly no treatment effect. We generated some pseudo-data with a small upward trend, nothing corresponding to an intervention, and some random variation such as would be expected in an experiment of this kind. We collected a few sets of 15 "observations" in this way, and chose a set that would best make our point, but several others were almost as good. We generated the simulated data using the equation $y = 5 + 0.2x$ with x taking values from 1 to 15 to give us data with a small upward trend, and then we added to each value a random number from the Normal distribution with mean zero and standard deviation 1.5.

First we examined the consequences of the response-guided approach. Our simulated data were supposed to be from a single-case AB design to evaluate the effectiveness of assertiveness training on frequency of contributions to group discussions by a shy student. The experiment will have 15 observations, and there must be a minimum of four in each phase. Baseline sessions will be continued until a stability criterion of four-in-a-row nearly equal scores is obtained, after which assertiveness training will be given. Table 6.1 shows the dataset we chose from several simulations. You can see that observations 2–5 are all pretty similar, so we can suppose the intervention is applied before observation 6. The phases are as shown in the third column, phase (1), of Table 6.1. If you look at the rest of the data you can see that the first five observations are all smaller than any later ones (Figure 6.1(a)). So it would be easy to believe on the basis of these data that the intervention did have the effect of increasing the scores, even though we know that there is no intervention at observation 6 or anywhere else in these simulated data.

Our next step was to examine the same data but this time supposing we had used randomization to select the intervention point. We chose a random number between 5 and 12 (we got 10) and supposed that this was the first observation in the intervention phase. The new phases are in the fourth column (phase (2)) of Table 6.1. Figure 6.1(b) shows the plot with the new phases, and we think few people looking at this would believe there was a treatment effect. Here it looks as if we have an upward trend that is not affected by the intervention. We performed a randomization

Table 6.1 Simulated Data to Demonstrate Bias

Limits	Data	Phase (1)	Phase (2)
15	3.80	0	0
4	4.96	0	0
4	4.80	0	0
	4.91	0	0
	4.99	0	0
	7.00	1	0
	6.73	1	0
	7.82	1	0
	7.30	1	0
	7.67	1	1
	6.53	1	1
	7.00	1	1
	8.93	1	1
	6.19	1	1
	5.89	1	1

test using the macro for the single-case AB design and phase (2) as the phase. The actual test statistic was 1.22, and the probability of a value at least as large was 0.74, a long way from significance. (Of course, with only eight possible intervention points, the smallest possible probability is 1/8 or 0.125, so significance at 5% would not be achievable.) So these data, generated entirely at random, make quite a convincing case for a treatment effect if you believe the intervention phase starts at observation 6, but show no treatment effect if you believe the intervention phase starts at observation 10 (or, in fact, at most other available points).

Use of a response-guided procedure to select an intervention point often gives us our best chance of finding a spurious effect, whether we use statistical or visual analysis. It is true, of course, that the data in Figures 6.1(a) and 6.1(b) were carefully selected from a number of datasets, generated using the same equation and random normal deviate, to provide a clear illustration of the argument for random determination of the intervention point. Not all such datasets were equally compelling, but it should not be assumed that misleading consequences of response-guided intervention are likely to be confined to carefully selected datasets.

An experimental test of response-guided bias

A small experiment was carried out to ascertain the effect of response-guided versus random determination of the intervention point on

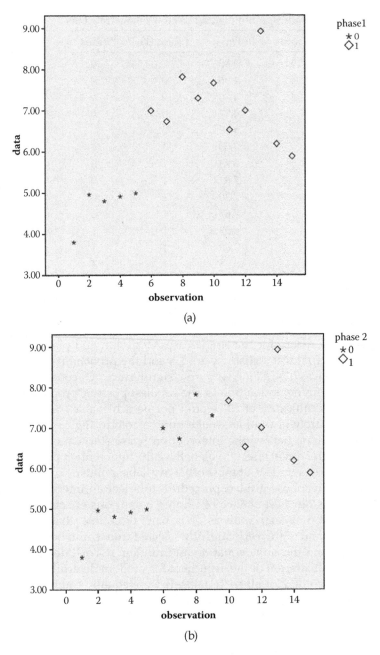

Figure 6.1 (a) Intervention phase starts at point 6. (b) Intervention phase starts at point 10.

frequency of incorrect inferences, using the same equation and random normal deviate to generate datasets (Todman & Dugard, 1999). Eighty graphs each with 15 observations were generated using the same equation and random deviate as in the example. In 50 of these graphs, it was possible to identify several fairly flat points in a row that could be used to designate an intervention point. Two copies of each of the 50 graphs were prepared, and a vertical line was drawn on each to indicate the intervention point. On one of each pair of copies, the intervention point followed immediately after the "flat points" to give a response-guided intervention point. On the other, the intervention point was randomly assigned to one of the sessions between session 5 and session 12, inclusive (so each phase had a minimum of four observations).

Twelve psychology students, moderately familiar with interpretation of graphical data, were each given the pile of 100 graphs in a different random order and asked to sort them into two piles, those showing an effect of treatment and those not showing an effect. The mean numbers of graphs sorted into the "effective treatment" pile were 33.0 (*sd* = 6.0) for those with the intervention following the flat points, and 11.4 (*sd* = 8.6) for those with randomly assigned intervention points. This difference was highly significant in a two-tailed related t test ($t = 9.84$, $df = 11$, $p < 0.001$), and the method of assignment of the intervention point accounted for 90% of the variance. Though the severity of the problem may vary with different baseline trends, degrees of random variability and serial correlation in the data, and the experience of the judges, our results are consistent with those reported by Franklin et al. (1996). It is difficult to resist the conclusion that response-guided assignment of treatment intervention points is indeed likely (as consideration of the logic of the procedure predicts) to result in more false positive inferences than would be the case using a randomization design and test.

Statistical consequences of response-guided experimentation

Apart from the internal validity problem occasioned by response-guided procedures in phase designs, which applies regardless of whether visual or statistical analysis is applied to the data, these procedures have the added disadvantage of ruling out the possibility of valid statistical analysis in many cases. We saw in Chapter 2 that some form of random procedure in the assignment of conditions to participants or observation times is a prerequisite for the use of randomization tests. Because these are the only statistical tests that are both valid and practical for some single-case designs (such as phase designs, unless there are enough observations for a time series analysis), the use of nonrandom, response-guided procedures in these designs effectively makes them nonamenable to statistical analysis.

Proponents of applied behavioral analysis may argue that the non-availability of valid statistics is of little consequence, visual analysis being always the method of choice because it is less sensitive than statistical analysis. This lack of sensitivity is desirable because it means that large (clinically significant) effects will be picked up and statistically significant, but clinically unimportant, effects will be excluded. But we have seen that the assumption that visual analysis is a more conservative procedure than statistical analysis is not supported by evidence.

Incomplete randomization

Nonrandomized classification variables

Random assignment of conditions to participants or observation occasions is an important requirement when we want to use randomization tests, just as it is when using ANOVA, t tests, and other parametric tests in large-n studies. However, in large-group designs, it is quite common for this requirement to be violated. Often there is something to be learned from large-n experiments even if random assignment is violated, as we discuss in the next paragraph. The purpose of this section is to consider whether anything may also be learned from applying a randomization test even if random assignment has not been properly done.

In large-n studies, classification variables, such as gender, age, and IQ, are frequently included as independent variables, though there is, of course, no question of levels of these variables being randomly assigned to subjects by the researcher. As Minium, King, and Bear (1993) made clear, studies lacking random assignment of the independent variable cannot correctly be called "experiments." When a statistically significant result is found, we can conclude that there was probably some systematic effect on the dependent variable, but we cannot safely infer that it was an effect of the classification variable because different levels of a variable such as gender are likely to be associated with differences on other variables such as socialization practices. However, this does not mean that nothing useful can be learned from designs using classification variables. Conclusions are necessarily cautious, but may at least indicate whether further work is justified.

Similarly, it may provide useful information to perform the randomization test calculations even when there has not been a random assignment of conditions. Edgington and Onghena (2007) described the following example. Researchers wish to compare urban and rural people on some physical fitness measure. Of course, there is no random assignment, but if we apply the one-way analysis, rearranging the "urban" and "rural" labels as if they were labels for randomly assigned experimental conditions, we will obtain the proportion of values in the reference set at least as large as the actual value. If this proportion is small, we may think it worth continuing to research this area even though explanations other than the difference between urban and rural living will be possible. If the proportion of the reference set is at least as large as the actual value is large, then probably we would not think the idea worth pursuing. Hence the application of a randomization test may help a researcher to decide whether to proceed with a line of investigation even if random assignment has not been used.

Here is another example, this time with a condition that will be randomly assigned to participants, and a classification variable. We are interested in a treatment for patients suffering chronic pain. Mindfulness meditation has been found to be useful in reducing disability scores (McCracken et al., 2007). However, programs that encourage mindfulness practice also encourage stretches, and there is some debate about how the two should be combined. Stretching prior to mindfulness practice may be more pleasant, but stretching after may allow the patient to be more responsive to their current pain level and less likely to overdo it. These effects might be different for neuropathic pain and musculoskeletal pain. So the two experimental conditions are stretches followed by meditation, and meditation followed by stretches, and these will be assigned at random to participants with the two kinds of pain. If we have equal numbers of participants in the four groups (two conditions and two kinds of pain), we could use the macro for the 2*2 factorial design to find the main effect of the experimental conditions. Although the kind of pain cannot be classed as a factor because the levels have not been assigned at random, we may get some indication whether we need to continue to allow for the kind of pain by looking at the probability associated with its "main effect." Even better, within each condition we could apply a one-way analysis (as we would to get simple effects in a proper factorial design) to get some idea of whether there is indeed some difference in the way patients with different kinds of pain respond or whether it would be reasonable to ignore this in future evaluations.

Ordinal predictions

There are two other related circumstances in which there may be a case for using a randomization test in the absence of a random assignment procedure in the design. One is the situation in which ordinal predictions are made for a dependent variable on the basis of classification variables. Here is an example. An educational psychologist suspects that problem behavior in the classroom may be related to failure to progress in reading. She asks a class teacher to name the six most difficult pupils in the class and obtains their scores on a standard reading test for their age. She asks the teacher to rank the children in order from least to most problem behavior. The psychologist's prediction is that the difficulty ranking will be the same as the reading score ranking. There are 6! or 720 possible orders for the difficulty ranks, so if the order is the same as the one for reading scores, we may think this provides some support for the psychologist's idea. Even if the orders are not identical but we apply the macro for order effects and find the test statistic in the top few percent of the reference set, we may still think it worth further investigation. There has been no random assignment here, and what we have observed is only an association. Just as when we use classification variables with classical statistical analysis, we can't deduce cause and effect from an association, but we may find useful clues in our search for greater understanding.

The second situation where we may get useful information by predicting an order in the absence of random assignment is a variant of the phase designs where phases can only have fixed lengths, so we cannot randomize the intervention points. Nevertheless, if we have an ABAB design with fixed-length phases, we may obtain some support if we have a hypothesis that predicts an order for the phase means that would not be accounted for by the lapse of time, practice, or boredom. Suppose, for example, that we predict B2 > B1 > A2 > A1. There are 4! = 24 possible arrangements of the data, and the smallest possible p value would be 0.042 if we had been able to apply A1, A2, B1, and B2 in random order. If the results are in the predicted order, then we may think we have an idea worth further investigation.

There may be other circumstances when it is reasonable to relax the random assignment requirement for carrying out a randomization test. It may, for example, be a sensible strategy for the analysis of pilot data or the analysis of existing data, where the analysis implications of failing to incorporate a random assignment procedure were not realized when the data were collected. In any case where a randomization test is applied to data obtained without random assignment, it should be made clear in reporting what was done, and the results must be interpreted with appropriate caution.

Exercises

1. Why do you need a list of a population from which you want to take a random sample?
2. What is the defining feature of a randomization design?
3. We are more likely to miss an effect in our experiment if our participants vary in a lot in ways that may affect results. But if we manage to choose a very similar group of participants and so increase our chance of observing an effect, what do we risk losing?

4. What is the main purpose of randomization?
5. In classical statistics, what is it that should provide external validity?
6. If you intend to rely on graphical analysis, why would you bother to randomize the intervention point in a phase design?
7. ANOVA is often described as robust, so why should you worry about the failure to use a random sample?
8. Are there occasions when you would consider using a randomization test even if there has been no random assignment?

chapter seven

Size and power

Introduction

Estimating the power of randomization tests is not always straightforward. Also, especially for phase designs, low power can be a problem. In this chapter, we consider ways to estimate power and also we review some of the ways in which power can be maximized. These are generally good experimental practice and apply to designs other than the randomization designs we are concerned with here. Phase designs and their special problems are discussed in the final section of the chapter. For these designs, effort spent on maximizing power is particularly important.

However, before we begin our consideration of power, we need to look at the significance level, p value, or α level for our tests. Statisticians use the term *size* for this probability that the null hypothesis is rejected when it is in fact true. Later in the chapter we also use the term size to help us to think clearly about power. But first, because our macros for implementing randomization tests have used random sampling of the reference set, as described at the end of Chapter 2, we need to look more closely at how this could affect α.

Estimating α by sampling the reference set

In Chapter 2 we explained that there are two ways to obtain the reference set: complete enumeration or random sampling. For some designs there are many millions of possible arrangements, and even when using a fast computer, obtaining the complete list and calculating the test statistic for each of them to get the reference set would be very time consuming. Also, although it is usually easy to work out how many arrangements are possible, in many cases making a list is surprisingly difficult. In all our macros, we have used the same method: We have taken a random sample with replacement of 2000 arrangements and used this to estimate the position in the reference set of our actual test statistic from the experiment. Now it is time for us to justify both our decision to use random sampling and the size of the sample.

In some cases, the number of possible arrangements is less than 2000, sometimes a lot less. This means that, in a random sample with replacement, many arrangements may be obtained more than once. If the number of possible arrangements is less than the sample size, the sample is said to be *saturated*. In what follows, it doesn't matter whether or not the sample is saturated; the results apply in all cases.

If we could list all possible arrangements and find the test statistic for each, so that we have the complete reference set, then by arranging the values in order we could see exactly the probability of values at least as extreme as our actual experimental one. This would be the significance level we would quote. If instead of a complete list we use a random sample of arrangements, then we need to know that the significance level we quote using the sample is close to what we would have obtained by using the complete list.

First suppose we want to use the 5% significance level, so we want to reject the null hypothesis (H_0) if the probability of obtaining an observed value of the test statistic at least as extreme as ours under H_0 is less than 0.05. If we use a random sample of arrangements instead of the complete list, we want to reject H_0 if we would have rejected it using the full list, and we want to accept it if we would have accepted it using the full list. Manly (2007) showed that a random sample of 1000 arrangements would be almost certain to achieve this unless the probability of obtaining an observed value of the test statistic at least as extreme as ours under H_0 is close to 0.05.

Our example for the single-case randomized blocks design is one where the probability of a result at least as extreme as ours if H_0 is true is close to 0.05. Running the macro several times is likely to produce probabilities just either side of the critical 0.05 value. In a case such as this, whether we are using a randomization test or a more conventional ANOVA, we would be reporting that our result was close to the 5% significance level, perhaps indicating that further work would be worthwhile.

In the macros we have used random samples of 2000 arrangements, which should usually be adequate if we are using the 5% significance level, though as in the example quoted above, there may still be some doubt about which side of 0.05 a borderline probability falls. However, what if we want to use the 1% significance level? In this case Manly showed that a random sample of 5000 arrangements will almost certainly bring us to the same conclusion as the complete list, unless the probability is close to 0.01.

If you want to change the number of arrangements in the random sample for any macro from 2000 to 5000, 1000, or indeed any other value, this is easy to do. We explain how to make this and other changes to the macros in Chapter 8.

Size and power: some terminology

Most users of statistical tests use the terms significance level, p value, or α level to denote the probability that the null hypothesis is rejected when it is in fact true. Rejecting the null hypothesis when it is true is a *Type 1 error*, so the significance level, *p* value, or α level is the probability of a Type 1 error. Among statisticians, α is referred to as the *size* of the test. So if we use the 5% significance level we are using a test of size 0.05. If an experimenter intends to use a statistical test of a null hypothesis, they should choose the size of the test before they begin the experiment. In practice this has never been the custom: An experimenter reports the highest significance level supported by the data. When a test statistic was calculated by hand, the result was referred to a table; and if it was significant at the 5% or 1% level, this would be reported. Now, test statistics are nearly always calculated by statistical software, and the exact probability of a result at least as extreme under H_0 is given as well, and often this is what is reported. So most people think of the probability as giving an indication of the strength of the evidence against H_0, rather than using it to decide whether or not H_0 should be rejected.

To think clearly about power, we need to think about the size of the test in the more formal way a statistician would prefer, but before we do that we can think of it in practical terms like this. We would like a perfect test for something like HIV. The null hypothesis is that the person does not have HIV. We want everyone who has HIV to be positive and everyone who does not have HIV to be negative on the test. In practice no such perfect tests exist: A few people without HIV will test positive (this is analogous to a Type 1 error), but we keep the probability of this as low as possible, say below 5%, to avoid frightening and treating people unnecessarily. Also, a few people who do have HIV will be negative (this is a *Type 2 error*, described below), and we would like the probability of this also to be low. The probability of declaring that a person without HIV has it is analogous to the size (or significance), and the probability of correctly detecting that a person has HIV is analogous to the power.

The size of the test is chosen by the experimenter before starting work, and it is the probability they are prepared to accept of making a Type 1 error. H_0 will be rejected if and only if the probability of a test statistic at least as extreme as the experimental one under H_0 is less than the chosen size of the test. In this formal scenario, a *Type 2 error* is failing to reject H_0 when it is in fact false. The probability of a Type 2 error is usually denoted by β. The *power* of the test is 1-β, the probability that we don't make a Type 2 error or do correctly reject H_0.

Unfortunately, although the size of a test can be chosen by the experimenter, the power is more problematical. The reason we can choose the size of a test is that H_0 is simple: It sets a specific value (usually zero) for a difference between means, a correlation, or whatever we are interested in. So if H_0 is true, it's easy to work out the probability of any experimental result. However, if H_0 is not true, it may be not true by a little or by a lot. If H_0 says the difference between two means is zero and the alternative says it is not zero, the difference could be only a bit different from zero, or it could be very large, or it could be anywhere in between. Assuming the difference is not zero, the probability of a significant result will depend on how large the difference is. A large difference is much more likely to give a significant result than a small one, so the power of the test depends on the size of the difference (the effect size).

The size we choose for the test also influences the power. If we decide we need a 1% significance level before we reject H_0, the test will be less powerful than if we settle for the 5% level. This is because to get a result that is significant at the 1% level, we need a more extreme value of the test statistic, so we are less likely to reject H_0. So, the power of a test depends on the size of the test and the effect size. It is also usually influenced by the number of participants or observations (n) – increasing the n usually increases the power. Much effort goes into trying to estimate the n needed to achieve a particular power for a given effect size and significance level, but before considering this we look at the ways in which power can be improved for any given n.

Maximizing power

In this section, we remind you of the ways in which power can be maximized. All these are just the best practice in experimental work, and they apply equally to randomization designs and more conventional ones.

Control of nuisance variables

People are extremely variable, and from the point of view of an experimenter, most of the ways they vary can be ascribed to *nuisance variables*, variables that are of no interest to the experimenter and that can mask any effect of different experimental conditions. Provided that participants have been randomly assigned to conditions, we can assume that the variability *within* conditions is caused by the random nuisance variables that distinguish our participants. But the larger the variability within conditions, the more plausible it becomes that this variability is responsible for any difference between means in the experimental conditions, so the larger experimental effect will be needed to enable rejection of H_0. If we can reduce the variability within conditions, then we have a better chance of detecting a real effect: The test will be more powerful. Working with a homogeneous group of participants may reduce within condition variability if we can make a good judgment about the ways in which we want the group to be homogeneous. Do we need a group with similar ages? The same sex? Similar work backgrounds? Similar symptoms? We need to look for homogeneity in variables that may influence what we are investigating. Of course, if we use a homogeneous group, our results may not generalize well, but if we find an effect, then it can be investigated in other homogeneous groups. This will often be a more efficient way forward than risking missing an effect by looking for it in a group that is so variable that we are likely to miss it.

When it is feasible to use repeated measures on the same participants, then we eliminate the differences among participants because they act as their own control. When repeated measures on the same participants are impractical, perhaps because of carry over effects, it may be possible to match participants on the basis of a single relevant variable. Our randomized blocks design could accommodate this. For instance, suppose we are investigating three methods of improving children's reading age. We could match children by reading age in blocks of three, and then apply each method at random to one child in each block of three. Rearrangement of the methods within blocks would be used to obtain the reference set for the randomization test, and the same macro would do the job. In either case, using repeated measures or matching on a relevant variable, the gain in power may be considerable.

Not all nuisance variables are those that distinguish participants. Other examples are variations between times of day or from day to day, or between observers or scorers. Some of these can be controlled by eliminating or minimizing the effects, as when stimuli are presented on a computer instead of by hand on flash cards, or reinforcement is always administered by the same person rather than by one of several. On other occasions, it may be preferable to control a nuisance variable by making it a factor in the experimental design. Our example for the single-case randomized blocks design uses this approach: Each day is a block because variation from day to day is a nuisance variable. When it is impractical to eliminate a random nuisance variable or to elevate it to the status of a factor in the design, it may be possible to control the nuisance variable statistically by treating it as a *covariate*. An analysis of covariance evaluates the effect of the independent variable after allowing for any effect of the covariate. We do not provide a macro for covariance analysis, but Edgington and Onghena (2007) did. They also explained what would be needed to extend our one-way design to include a covariate.

Of course, random nuisance variables are abundant in real-world environments, and controlling them always runs the risk of reducing the external validity of experiments. In the last resort, we are interested in the effects that variables have in natural environments. However, if we find a significant effect in a well-controlled laboratory setting or in a homogeneous group of participants, we may be encouraged to explore its effect in less controlled settings.

Increasing reliability of measurements

Another way of looking at the variability within conditions is in terms of the unreliability of measurements. Sometimes, variability within conditions is not due to the effects of other variables; it is just that the measuring instrument is inconsistent. If we are concerned that our bathroom scales give us different answers as we repeatedly step on and off, we assume that the problem is with the scales rather than with some other random variable. So, if we are using a rating scale to measure our dependent variable, and it has a low reliability, we would probably be wasting our time looking for random nuisance variables to control. If it were possible to improve the reliability of our measuring instrument, the power of our test should increase as the variability of measurements within a condition decreases. One way of increasing the reliability of measurement is to increase the number of measurements taken for each observation period, and another is to increase the number of independent observers. In terms of ratings, we can have more raters or more ratings per rater. There is a useful chapter by Primavera, Allison, and Alfonso (1997) in which they discussed methods for promoting the reliability of measurements.

Maximizing effect size

In general, we use the term *effect* for a measure of the change produced by our experimental manipulation. It's useful to have a measure of effect size that does not depend on the units of measurement. For example, instead of the difference between two means we might use the difference divided by the standard deviation estimated from all the measurements. Cohen (1988) suggested that using this measure of effect size, 0.2 would be a small effect, 0.5 would be medium, and 0.8 would be a large effect. So, in these terms, a large effect is one where the difference between means is 0.8 of the standard deviation. There is an analogous measure for more than two means. So although we can choose the size of test to use, the power depends on the effect size.

We can influence the size of the effect by the levels we choose for the independent variable. In our example for the small-group one-way design, we were looking for differences among the practice hours needed to learn to use different communication aids. We had four aids, and we didn't specify how they differed. If they were fairly similar and differ only in insignificant details, the experimental effect may be quite small and the power of our experiment rather low. But if we only compare two aids, one the very latest high-tech device and the other a rather early model, then we may find a much larger effect and our experiment will be correspondingly powerful. Likewise, when we give the mindfulness training to the pain sufferer in the single-case AB example, we can give really intensive training, the very best available, or we can give a single short session and keep the cost down. The effect may be larger and our experiment more powerful if we deliver the training in the most effective way we can.

Of course, when we select extreme values for our levels of the independent variable, we run the risk that the effect does not apply to most cases that would be encountered in reality. Clearly, there is a balance to be struck here. In the early stages of exploring the efficacy of a novel treatment, we might well be concerned not to miss a real effect, so increasing power by maximizing the intervention may make sense. In later research into a promising treatment, we will probably be more concerned to explore the robustness of its effects when it is administered in a more economical way. (This would be Phase V in Robey's model of the research process described in Chapter 1.)

The choice of values for fixed features of an experiment may also influence effect size. For example, consider a single-case study with two randomized treatments to compare the effects of contingent and noncontingent reinforcement on the frequency of positive self-statements. The single-case randomized blocks design could be used. Choice of different lengths of observation period, different intervals between treatment occasions, or different intervals after reinforcement sessions before commencement of observation periods would all be likely to influence effect size. For example, in repeated measures designs, longer *washout* intervals between treatments are likely to result in larger effect sizes.

Increasing precision of prediction

When using the familiar *t* test for a difference between means, if our alternative hypothesis specifies the direction of any difference, then the one-tailed test is more powerful than the two-tailed test we would use for an alternative that doesn't specify direction. Similarly, if we specify in advance a few comparisons to make after performing an ANOVA, the available tests are more powerful than the Scheffé test, which allows for post hoc comparisons of subsets of levels using contrasts. Generally, we can use a more powerful test for a more precise prediction. This is also generally true for randomization tests. However, a one-tailed test is not necessarily more powerful than a two-tailed one for phase designs.

Opinion about the desirability of using one-tailed tests is divided. Our view is that this is no less acceptable than making any other designed comparison within sets of means following formulation of an a priori hypothesis. The critical requirements are that the hypothesis be formulated before data are collected and obtained differences in the nonpredicted direction result in a "not statistically significant" decision.

Using a directional alternative and a one-tailed test is an example of making an ordinal prediction (A > B instead of A ≠ B). Ordinal predictions of any degree of complexity may be made. The more specific the prediction, the greater will be the power of the test to detect that precise effect, but its power to detect *near misses* (a slightly different order than that predicted) becomes lower. Particularly with sparse data (which is not uncommon with single-case designs), it may be worthwhile considering whether power could be increased by making ordinal predictions (in which case it may be possible to use our design to test order effects).

Power of randomization tests

For randomization tests that are analogs of ANOVA or other classical tests, if the assumptions needed for the classical test are satisfied, then the size of the randomization test is similar to that for the corresponding classical test (Manly, 2007). It might be expected that in these cases, the power of the randomization test is also similar to that of the classical test, and Manly quoted several studies that support this view. Estimating power from a classical test is discussed further below.

One important assumption for classical tests is the independence of observations. Single-case designs, and especially phase designs, may be subject to serial correlation in the data. We consider the power of phase designs below. For a review of the effects of serial correlation in single-case designs, see Matyas and Greenwood (1996). We show how to check for serial correlation in Appendix 1, and in Chapter 3 we suggest how to keep it low.

Another complication for power considerations is that, starting with the same basic design, different randomization procedures are possible, each of which will have a different set of possible data arrangements associated with it. This means that the power of a randomization test will vary with the randomization procedure used. We discussed different randomization procedures in Chapter 4 for our single-case one-way design example. Our design (and the macro) takes the number of observations in each condition as fixed (we had three observations in each of three conditions). An alternative design would allow the number of observations in each condition to be determined by the randomization process. It would still be a one-way design, but the set of possible arrangements and so the reference set would be different. Because rejection of the null hypothesis depends on the position of the test statistic in the ordered reference set, a different reference set is likely to give a different probability of rejection and so a different power.

Estimating power from a classical test

In cases where it is reasonable to estimate the power of a randomization test from that of a corresponding classical test, we have a deterministic system comprising *power*, *α-level*, *effect size*, and *sample size* (usually number of participants). If we know the values of any three, the value of the fourth can be determined. Usually, we want to know one of two things. Before conducting an experiment, we may want to know how many participants we need to ensure a specified power, given values for α and a critical effect size. After conducting an experiment in which we failed to find a significant effect, we may want to know what the power of the test was, given the number of participants included in our design. Alternatively, after an experiment has been conducted, by either ourselves or others, we may want to know the power of the test in order to decide how many participants to use in an experiment involving similar variables.

First, we must decide on a value for α (usually 0.05 or 0.01), bearing in mind that a low value for α will make it harder to achieve a high power for the test for a fixed sample size. Then we must decide on a critical value for effect size: What is the effect size that is sufficiently important to us that we really do not want to miss it? In the absence of any indications from previous related research or clinical criteria, one of Cohen's values for high, medium, or low effect size, which were described in this chapter, may be selected. If the intention is to determine how many participants are needed to achieve a given power, then the level of power needs to be set, bearing in mind that convention has it that a power of 0.8 is considered acceptable and a power of 0.9 is considered good. The final step is to use the values of α, effect size, and power to find *n* by calculation, reading its value from a table or a graph, or obtaining it from a computer package, bearing in mind that the value of *n* is the number of participants needed for *each* condition. SPSS SamplePower© (details on the SPSS Web site) is an attractive option for this last step.

If the intention is to determine the power for a given number of participants, the α level and effect size need to be set as before, and the number (*n*) of participants per condition must be known. In this case, the final step is to use the values of α, effect size and *n* to obtain a value for power, using any of the methods referred to above.

Single-case analogs of ANOVA

Power considerations are most straightforward for those single-case designs that are analogs of large-*n* designs for which power functions are available. For the single-case one-way design, treatments are randomly assigned to observation times, and the number of observations per treatment is analogous to the number of subjects per treatment in a large-n design where there is random assignment of treatments to participants. Where an equivalent large-n design exists, the power of a randomization test can be estimated using the power function for a test that would be applied to the large-n design. Edgington (1969) provided an analytic proof of this, and Onghena (1994) confirmed it empirically except for small group sizes. Our view is that power calculations should be regarded as very approximate estimates for the equivalent randomization test.

Phase designs

A phase design may be the design of last resort in the investigation of an intervention that cannot be randomly assigned to observation periods or participants. Unfortunately, the power of phase designs is generally quite low. Ferron and Ware (1995) investigated several single-case designs: an AB design with 30 observations, an ABAB design with 32 observations, and a multiple baseline AB design with 15 observations on each of four participants. Six effect sizes (from no effect to 1.4 standard deviations) and four levels of serial correlation were studied. Even with the largest effect size of 1.4, power estimates were generally low (recall that an effect size of 0.8 is classed as large by Cohen). They found low power (less than 0.5) even for an effect size as large as 1.4 with no serial correlation present. With positive serial correlation, power was even lower. This is quite discouraging, and shows how important it is to maximize power in any way possible when using a phase design.

Ferron and Sentovich (2002) estimated the power for a multiple baseline design with intervention points randomly assigned, for effect sizes 0, 0.5, 1.0, 1.5, and 2.0. They studied series lengths 10, 20, and 30 and serial correlations 0, 0.1, 0.2, 0.3, 0.4, and 0.5. They found power was usually low for effect sizes 0.5 and 1.0, but often adequate (> 0.8) for effect sizes 1.5 and 2.0. This again emphasizes the importance of maximizing the effect size and also using any other available method to increase power.

Common sense and knowledge of classical tests might suggest that we can increase the power of a phase design by increasing the length of the observation series. Onghena (1994) noted an interesting contradiction to the assumption that more observations would result in more power. Here is his example. Suppose we have 29 observation periods with the minimum number of observations per phase set at 5. There will be 20 possible intervention points, and to reject the null hypothesis at the 5% level we need the actual test statistic to be more extreme than any of the other arrangement statistics. An increase in number of observations from 29 to

39 would mean 30 possible intervention points. However, to achieve 5% significance we would still only be able to reject the null hypothesis if the actual test statistic was more extreme than any of the other arrangement statistics, because 2/30 >0.05. In this case, our rejection region would be 1/30 instead of 1/20 of the possible results, a smaller proportion of the sample space than in the case with only 29 observations, so power would be reduced. Of course, α would also be reduced from 0.05 to 1/30 or 0.03, but this gain would probably be of no interest, so the overall effect of increasing the number of observations from 29 to 39 would be to reduce the power while leaving the usable α level the same.

It was also apparent from Onghena's simulations that virtually no gain in power could be expected for the AB design as a result of making a directional prediction. To put things into perspective, he found that to achieve a power of 0.8 for an effect size of 0.8 and with α set at 0.05, an AB design with randomized assignment of the intervention point would require 10 times as many observations as a randomized treatment design.

Considering the internal validity limitations of the AB design along with its unimpressive power, it seems necessary to question the usefulness of this frequently used design. It does seem, at least, that its usefulness may be limited to very large effect sizes. This fits with the intuitions of applied behavior researchers, who stress the importance of seeking large (clinically significant) effects in phase studies of this kind. It seems, however, that their statistical intuitions are mistaken when they assume that statistical analysis of single-case phase data is likely to lead to finding too many statistically significant, but clinically trivial, effects. On the contrary, it seems quite likely that, with the number of observations typically used, none but the largest effects will be picked up. The sensitivity of phase designs with randomly assigned intervention point(s) may be increased by the addition of a reversal phase or by means of the inclusion of multiple baselines. The Ferron and Sentovich work mentioned above (2002) suggests that at least for really large effects, power may be adequate in multiple baseline designs.

Exercises

1. Why is it often necessary to estimate where a test statistic falls in the reference set by random sampling instead of calculating all values in the reference set?
2. Why might you want to edit our macros to increase the size of the sample from the reference set from 2000 to something larger?
3. What do statisticians mean by the "size" of a test? What determines the size of a test?

4. What do we mean by the "power" of a test? What determines the power of a test?
5. How might increasing the power reduce the external validity?
6. Why might increasing power at the expense of external validity be a good way to proceed?
7. Phase designs generally have rather low power, so why use them?
8. Are phase designs likely to pick up effects that are clinically insignificant?

chapter eight

Going further

Introduction

This book offers randomization test macros for just a few designs, and you may by now be wondering why there are not more, or indeed why statistical software such as SPSS does not offer them. When we use the usual parametric and nonparametric statistical tests, we are making use of the fact that if the null hypothesis is true, it is possible to calculate the distribution of the test statistic. The distributions of most of the commonly used test statistics were tabulated decades ago. In order to see how probable is the value of the test statistic we obtained from our experiment, we only have to consult a table. In fact, when using software such as SPSS, we do not even need to do that because the probability under the null hypothesis of a value at least as extreme as the one we obtained is given with the test statistic. In contrast, to use a randomization test, we have to find the values in the reference set ourselves. Whether we list and calculate every value in the reference set, or use a sampling method as in our macros, obtaining the reference set for comparison with our experimental value is not a process that can be fully generalized. So each design needs its own macro or other software. If you want to use a design that does not fit one of our macros, you could see if there is other software that will support the analysis of your chosen design. In the "Other Sources of Software for Randomization Tests" section of this chapter, we briefly list some sources of software other than our macros. Another option is to modify one of our macros to fit your design. The penultimate section in this chapter explains how you can do this.

Other sources of software for randomization tests

A comprehensive list of free and commercial software is given by Edgington and Onghena (2007). The following list gives details of software to accompany books we have referenced, along with a brief note on the exact tests available in SPSS.

RT4Win

Randomization tests for windows (RT4Win) began as a suite of Fortran programs initially developed by Edgington for the first edition of *Randomization Tests* (1980). Many more designs are available than we provide with our macros. In the fourth edition (2007) of the book, coauthored with Onghena, there is a CD that contains RT4Win, now running on Windows and including tests for one-way and repeated measures ANOVA, independent and correlated *t*, and product moment ρ, all with random sampling with replacement or complete listing of the reference set. There are also trend tests, matching tests, and tests of main effects with random sampling of the reference set. The Fortran source code is also included as a Word document. Data can be entered on screen (there are clear instructions) or from a file. The book contains advice for modifying the source code and adapting it to write your own programs.

Single-case randomization tests (SCRT)

This is a package originally developed by Onghena and Van Damme (1994), and extended by Bulté and Ongehena (2008, 2009, 2011) and Bulté, Van Den Noortgate, and Onghena (2010). It now includes AB, ABA, ABAB, completely randomized, alternating treatments, randomized block, and multiple baseline designs.

The latest version of the SCRT software can be obtained free from http://ppw.kuleuven.be/cmes/SCRT-R.html. The scripts provided on this webpage are designed for use with R, which is the open-source implementation of the S-PLUS language. R is a free software environment for statistical computing and graphics. It compiles and runs on a wide variety of UNIX platforms, Windows, and MacOS. The most important advantage is that it can be downloaded free from the Comprehensive R Archive Network (CRAN) Web site, http://cran.r-project.org.

SCRT is also available on the CD that accompanies Edgington and Onghena (2007), with instructions in a *readme* file. Data can be entered on screen or from a file.

Howell's resampling programs

The Web site http://www.uvm.edu/~dhowell/StatPages/Resampling/Resampling.html gives details of software developed by David Howell. It can be downloaded free. There are also pages of text explaining randomization and bootstrap tests. Howell (2010) included a section on randomization and bootstrap tests.

Manly's RT software

Software to accompany Bryan Manly's book (Manly, 2007) has been written by him and can be purchased from http://www.west-inc.com/computer.php. Scroll down the page to the "RT" section. A trial version is available free for 30 days. The book appears in "Further Reading" in this chapter and has been referenced previously.

SPSS exact tests

In SPSS, the dialog box for **Analyze > Descriptive statistics > Crosstabs** has an **Exact** button, and there is also one in the dialog boxes for the non-parametric tests. These exact tests are randomization tests for which the usual χ^2 (chi-square) test and other nonparametric tests are approximations that give correct probabilities of Type 1 errors when large samples are used. However, most nonparametric tests use ranks rather than the original observations, and so some information is lost, especially if there are ties, so exact tests that use all of the information are usually preferable. Here is an example using our example data for the one-way small-group design. The Kruskal-Wallis test for differences among means from several independent samples uses just the ranks of the observations. Our example (Table 4.2) has 10 observations with several ties. Replacing the observations by their ranks, we have Table 8.1.

Using SPSS to obtain the exact version of the Kruskal-Wallis test (**Analyze > Nonparametric tests > K independent samples** and click the **Exact** button) on the data from Table 4.2 or the version with ranks in Table 8.1, we get SPSS Output 8.1. If we had not used the exact test and instead had used the chi-square large-sample approximation, we would

Table 8.1 Ranks for Small-Group One-Way Design Data

Data	Condition
3.5	1
3.5	1
1.0	2
3.5	2
6.5	3
3.5	3
6.5	3
10.0	4
8.5	4
8.5	4

Test Statistics[a,b]

	data
Chi-Square	7.750
df	3
Asymp. Sig.	.051
Exact Sig.	.007
Point Probability	.002

a. Kruskal-Wallis Test

b. Grouping Variable: condition

Figure 8.1 SPSS Output 8.1. Kruskal-Wallis test on data from Table 4.2 or Table 8.1.

have said that our data just failed to reach the 5% significance level. The chi-square value in the first row of Figure 8.1 *SPSS Output 8.1* is 7.750, but the 5% critical value for χ^2 with 3 degrees of freedom is 7.815. The value 7.750 has a probability of 0.051 (Asymp. Sig. in Figure 8.1 *SPSS Output 8.1*), just too high for significance at 5%. The asymptotic significance is the large sample approximation mentioned at the start of this section. The exact test gives the exact significance as 0.007. Our randomization test applied to the data in Table 4.2 (SPSS Output 5.2) gave a probability of 0.006 of a result as extreme as ours under the null hypothesis. Another run gave a probability of 0.005. We applied the randomization test to the ranks in Table 8.1 and got probabilities of 0.007 and 0.009 on two runs. In general, because the use of ranks rather than original data loses information (especially if there are ties), we expect that the randomization tests applied to original data will be more powerful than SPSS exact tests based on ranks. Similarly, when numbers are small, exact tests based on ranks are likely to be more powerful than large-sample approximations.

Writing your own macros: some general advice

If you want to try writing your own macros, a good starting point is one of the appendices (see Appendix 2 for SPSS and Appendix 3 for Excel). We have explained the techniques used and annotated each macro, but you will still find it quite an effort to understand, especially the sections that do the rearrangements.

To do the rearrangements, we always need to obtain random variables in particular ranges. We showed easy ways to do that in SPSS and Excel in Appendix 1, so you may wonder why it should be hard to do in the macros. To take the phase designs first, the problem there is mainly with the ABA designs, where the range for the withdrawal point depends on the intervention point. So we have to work out how many possible intervention–withdrawal pairs there are and list them. For each rearrangement, we use a random number to choose a pair.

For the other designs, we usually need to rearrange the observations, perhaps within blocks or levels of another factor. For SPSS, we start with the first observation and choose at random one to change places with it. Then we do the same with the next observation, using the observations below it in the list. So we need a succession of random numbers in a range that is reduced by one at each step. This process has to be enclosed in a loop to obtain 2000 rearrangements. It's certainly possible to do these operations, but it may take you nearly as much effort to understand them as it took us to get them working. In Excel, we can usually make a rearrangement by making a list of random numbers and then sorting the data by the random numbers. This has to be done for every rearrangement. The reward for the effort of understanding these steps is the ability to write new macros yourself.

The best way to start writing a new macro is to see what you can reuse from those we list in the appendices. While we were working on this book, a user of the first edition asked us how to analyze a design with several participants each of whom had received two conditions in random order. This would be our small-group repeated measures design with two conditions, except that the participants did not receive each condition only once: They received them five times each, arranged in random order over 10 observation periods. We did not have a macro to deal with this, but thought we could produce one, and we show you what we did in the next section of this chapter. We called the new design "A small-group repeated-measures design with replicates."

Using parts of our macros to write one of your own: an example

The new design we wanted, with each participant receiving two conditions on several occasions, has some similarities to the two-way factorial. Think of factor 1: There are several observations on each of two levels in level 1 of factor 2, and again in level 2 of factor 2. If we only had two participants, perhaps we could think of each participant as like a level of factor 2. But we have to see if we can adapt the macro to allow more than two participants.

When we look at the rearrangement process for the factorial design, we see that to get the main effect of factor 1, we have to rearrange the observations within each level of factor 2. In the new design, we need to rearrange the observations within each participant to find out whether there is any difference between the two conditions. So it looks as if we could use much of the factorial design, if only we could make it work with more than two levels of factor 2, which would give us the option of more than two participants.

This was how we began to work on the problem. The following paragraphs take you with us through the process of taking a piece of the
two-way factorial macro and using it as the basis for a new one, first in
SPSS and then in Excel. To get the most from this, you should first go to
Appendix 2 or 3 and understand as well as you can the macros for the
one-way design, the one-way with two conditions, and the two-way factorial. The new macro we developed as described below became the one for
the small-group repeated-measures design with replicates, and you can
see our example data in Table 4.7.

We show the SPSS version followed by Excel, so you need to read only
the one for your chosen package.

The SPSS version

The two-way factorial macro is in two parts, with the first part dealing
with factor 1. In our new design, the two conditions will replace the two
levels of factor 1, and the participants will replace factor 2. We shall only
reuse the first part of the factorial design macro.

We obtain the reference set for the factor 1 main effect by rearranging
the observations within each level of factor 2. To solve the new problem,
we would need to rearrange the observations within each participant. We
have only two conditions, just as we had only two levels of factor 1, but
we want to be able to use more than two participants, so we will have to
modify the first part of the two-way factorial macro so that the levels of
factor 2 are replaced by participant numbers and we need to allow more
than 2.

The datasheet for the two-way factorial (Tables 4.8 and 4.9) just has the
total number of observations in the first column. Because each combination of factor levels has to have the same number of observations, the total
number of observations is a multiple of four, and from it we can work out
how many observations are at each level of factor 1. For the new design,
we need more information in column 1 of the datasheet because we may
have more than two participants.

We have to tell the macro how many participants there are, as well as
how many observations on each. In the LIMITS column, we decided to put
first the number of participants, then the number of observations on each
participant (we are assuming we have the same number in each condition
and the same for each participant). From these two numbers, anything
else needed can easily be calculated, but we need to alter the few lines
of the macro that read the data. Here are the first few lines of the new
macro. As you can see if you check the factorial design in Appendix 2,
we have replaced the names FACTOR2 with CONDITION and FACTOR2 with

PARTICIPANT in the DATA matrix. From the LIMITS column, we have taken the number of participants (NCASE) and the number of observations per participant (NSWAPS) and from these calculated the number of observations (multiply participants by observations per participant and get NOBS). At the start of the factorial macro, we sorted the data by levels of factor 2. For the new macro, we are assuming the data are correctly arranged as in Table 4.7, and we do not include a sort.

```
set mxloops 5000.
matrix.
get limits/variables=limits/missing=omit.
get data/variables data condition participant/missing omit.
compute ncase=limits(1).
compute nswaps=limits(2).
compute nobs=ncase*nswaps.
```

Once we have obtained the data from the datasheet, the next job is to obtain the test statistic for the actual experiment. Because we have only two conditions, we will use the difference between condition means. A directional alternative and a one-tailed test will be possible, and if this is to be used then the macro assumes the condition coded 2 is the one predicted to have the higher mean. This is just as in the factorial design, and we obtain the test statistic in exactly the same way. The number of observations in each condition is half the total number of observations, and we divide the totals by this to get the condition means. In the factorial design, we divided by twice the number of replicates, which amounts to the same thing because factor 2 also had two levels. Here are the lines to obtain and print the test statistic in the new macro.

```
compute total={0,0}.
loop obs=1 to nobs.
compute total(data(obs,2))=total(data(obs,2))+data(obs,1).
end loop.
compute test1=(total(2)-total(1))/(nobs/2).
print test1/title="test statistic".
```

Next we prepare to do the rearrangements. We set the number of rearrangements, make a matrix to receive the test statistics obtained from them, put the value from the actual experiment in the first place, and start the arrangements loop, all exactly as in the factorial and indeed other designs. Here are the lines.

```
compute nperm=2001.
compute results=uniform(nperm,1).
compute results(1,1)=test1-test1/1000000.
loop perm=2 to nperm.
```

Now we have to rearrange observations within participants, so we need a loop to take us through participants one by one. This line starts it off. (In the factorial, we had only two levels of factor 2, so the command was loop fac2 = 1 to 2.)

```
loop case = 1 to ncase.
```

Within each participant, we have to rearrange the observations. We have NSWAPS observations for each participant, and we rearrange them using exactly the same method as we used to rearrange the NSWAPS observations at each level of factor 2. Here are the lines.

```
loop n= 1 to nswaps.
compute k=trunc(uniform(1,1)*(nswaps-n+1))+n+nswaps*(case-1).
compute obs=n+nswaps*(case-1).
compute temp=data(obs,1).
compute data(obs,1)=data(k,1).
compute data(k,1)=temp.
end loop.
```

Another end loop command closes the loop taking us through the participants. Now we need the test statistic for this arrangement. We calculate it in exactly the same way as we did the one for the actual experiment, and put it in the next place in the RESULTS matrix. Here are the lines.

```
compute total={0,0}.
loop obs=1 to nobs.
compute total(data(obs,2))=total(data(obs,2))+data(obs,1).
end loop.
compute test1=(total(2)-total(1))/(nobs/2).
compute results(perm,1)=test1.
```

Another end loop command closes the loop taking us through the 2000 rearrangements. The remainder of the macro is just the same as for the factorial and other designs where a one-tailed test is an option. Here it is for reference.

```
compute absres=abs(results).
compute pos1=0.
compute pos2=0.
loop k=2 to nperm.
do if results(k,1)>=results(1,1).
compute pos1=pos1+1.
end if.
do if absres(k,1)>=absres(1,1).
compute pos2=pos2+1.
end if.
end loop.
print pos1/title="count of arrangement statistics at least as large".
compute prob1=(pos1+1)/nperm.
```

```
print prob1/title="one tail probability".
print pos2/title="count of arrangement statistics at least as large
  in abs value as abs(test)".
compute prob2=(pos2+1)/nperm.
print prob2/title="two tail probability".
end matrix.
```

So the alterations to the part of the factorial macro that obtains the main effect of factor 1 are actually pretty trivial. We needed extra information in the first column of the datasheet, and we needed to loop from 1 to ncase when working through participants, whereas we needed to loop only from 1 to 2 when working through levels of factor 2.

Suppose we wanted a two-way factorial design with more than two levels of the factors. Of course, a one-tailed test would not then be an option, and we would have to use a different test statistic, the RSS perhaps. But by using parts of the one-way macro and most of the factorial macro, this would probably not be very hard to do. You may like to try it yourself.

The Excel version

The two-way factorial macro has blocks of code to deal with factor 1 and factor 2, and mostly we can get what we want by lifting out the factor 1 block. For the factorial macro, we had only the total number of observations in column A, but this won't do now that we need to give the number of participants. We decided that the first number in A would be the number of participants, and the second would be the number of observations per participant, so the total number of observations will be obtained by multiplying these. The first part of the factorial macro clears the columns to be used, reads column A, sets the last row of data, and sorts the data into order by factor 2 levels. We omit the sort in the new macro, assuming the data are correctly arranged as in Table 4.7.

In the new macro, we just need to read A3 as well as A2 and use them to get the total number of observations and hence the last data row. Here is the new version, with A2 called NCASE and A3 called NPERCASE.

```
Columns("E:M").ClearContents
Dim j As Integer
Dim lastcase$
Dim npercase$
Dim lastobs$
lastcase = Range("A2")
npercase = Range("A3")
lastobs = lastcase * npercase
Dim lastrow$
lastrow$ = lastobs + 1
```

The next set of instructions makes a copy of the observations that will then be rearranged within participants (or, in the factorial version, within levels of factor 2). Here it is in the new version.

```
Range("B2:B" & lastrow$).Select
Selection.Copy
Range("E2").Select
ActiveSheet.Paste
```

Now we need to do the rearrangements. Start by setting the number at 2000. Then put a set of random numbers in column F and sort the copied data in column E according to the random numbers in F. Once again, the original version needs no change because the process works just as well even if column D has codes for more than two participants.

```
For j = 1 To 2000
Range("F2").Select
ActiveCell.FormulaR1C1 = "=RAND()+RC[-2]"
Selection.AutoFill Destination:=Range("F2:F" & lastrow$), _
Type:=xlFillDefault
Range("E2:F" & lastrow$).Select
Selection.Sort Key1:=Range("F2"), Order1:=xlAscending, _
Header:=xlGuess, OrderCustom:=1, MatchCase:=False, _
Orientation:=xlTopToBottom
```

Now, for the rearranged observations, we need the difference between condition 2 and condition 1 means. This can be obtained in exactly the same way as the difference between factor 1 level means. We can use the original code just as it stands except that we need to divide by R2C1*R3C1 in the last line, this being the total number of observations, which for the factorial was in A2. Here is the version for the new macro.

```
Range("G2").Select
ActiveCell.FormulaR1C1 = "=(RC[-2]*(RC[-4]-1.5)*2)"
Selection.AutoFill Destination:=Range("G2:G" & lastrow$)
Range("H2").Select
ActiveCell.FormulaR1C1 = "=2*SUM(C[-1])/(R2C1*R3C1)"
```

The test statistic for the rearranged data must be stored, and then we can do the next arrangement. The process continues until all 2000 rearrangements have been done. Here is the original code for the factorial macro, and we can use it just as it stands. The Next command at the end here sends us to the next rearrangement.

```
Selection.Copy
Range("I2").Select
Selection.Insert Shift:=xlDown
Selection.PasteSpecial Paste:=xlValues
Next
```

The original macro now goes on to deal with factor 2, but we can ignore all that and go to the final part where we obtain the actual test statistics and probabilities for one- and two-tailed tests. Here is the bit where we set the last row of arrangement statistics and put the absolute values of the test statistics calculated from the rearrangements into the next empty column. In the new macro, the next empty column is J (it was O in the factorial version).

```
lastj$ = j + 1
Range("J2").Select
ActiveCell.FormulaR1C1 = "=ABS(C[-1])"
Selection.AutoFill Destination:=Range("J2:J" & lastj$)
```

Now we want to find the test statistic for the actual data and its absolute value for the two-tailed test. The next empty columns were Q and R in the factorial version, but for the new version we can use columns K and L. From K, we have to count back 9 columns to the actual data in column B and 8 to the conditions in column C. (The factorial version had to count back 15 and 14 from column Q.) We also need to remember that to get the number of observations for obtaining the mean, we have to multiply the numbers in column A and divide that by 2. Here is the new version.

```
Range("K2").Select
ActiveCell.FormulaR1C1 = "=(RC[-9]*(RC[-8]-1.5)*2)"
Selection.AutoFill Destination:=Range("K2:K" & lastrow$)
Range("L2").Select
ActiveCell.FormulaR1C1 = "=2*SUM(C[-1])/(R2C1*R3C1)"
Range("L3").Select
ActiveCell.FormulaR1C1 = "=ABS(R[-1]C)"
```

Now we have to count the number of values in the reference set that are at least as large as the actual test statistic and divide by 2001 to get the one-tailed probability. The results go into the next empty column, M (U in the factorial version). Our actual test statistic is in the previous column L (count back 1). To count the reference set values that are at least as large, we have to count back 4 columns to I, where we stored the test statistics from the rearrangements. So here is the new version.

```
Range("M2").Select
ActiveCell.FormulaR1C1 = "=RC[-1]"
Range("M3").Select
ActiveCell.FormulaR1C1 = "=COUNTIF(C[-4]:C[-4],"">=""&R[-1]C)"
Range("M4").Select
ActiveCell.FormulaR1C1 = "=(R[-1]C+1)/(2000+1)"
```

Now we just have to do the same calculations using absolute values to get the two-tailed probability. Here is the version for the new macro.

Notice that as absolute values are in column J, we count back three columns from M to do the comparisons.

```
Range("M5").Select
ActiveCell.FormulaR1C1 = "=R[-2]C[-1]"
Range("M6").Select
ActiveCell.FormulaR1C1 = "=COUNTIF(C[-3]:C[-3],""">=""&R[-1]C)"
Range("M7").Select
ActiveCell.FormulaR1C1 = "=(R[-1]C+1)/(2000+1)"
End Sub
```

The changes we had to make to the first part of the factorial macro to get the new one were not hard to do. Suppose we wanted a two-way factorial design with more than two levels of the factors. Of course, a one-tailed test would not then be an option, and we would have to use a different test statistic, the RSS perhaps. But by using parts of the one-way macro and most of the factorial macro, this would probably not be very hard to do. You may like to try it yourself.

Further reading

For those who want to learn more about randomization tests, Eugene Edgington's *Randomization Tests* is essential reading. The fourth edition, coauthored with Patrick Onghena (2007), includes a CD, referred to in the section on other software in this chapter. This book is essential reading for anyone wishing to know more about the subject and includes many more designs than we cover here. In addition, there is an excellent discussion of the principles and practice of randomization. The authors argued that for most experimenters, the random sample is a fiction, and that the legitimacy of the commonly used classical tests depends on the fact that they approximate randomization tests. There is an excellent chapter on validity and a comprehensive discussion of the available ways to maximize power. The final sections contain a guide to the programs on the CD and a list of other available software. We hope our book helps you to get your toes in the water, but Edgington and Onghena will enable you to swim.

The other text to read if you really want to know about randomization tests is Bryan Manly's *Randomization, Bootstrap and Monte Carlo Methods in Biology*, now in its third edition (2007). As the title suggests, this book covers more than randomization tests, which can be seen as a special case of the Monte Carlo method. The bootstrap method of Manly's title can also be explored in Efron (1982). It exploits the idea that if we have a random sample from a population, then if we know nothing else about that population we can use the sample values to estimate a population distribution. The name suggests we are pulling ourselves up by the bootstraps. Manly's book has good explanations and a rich collection of examples (and references to many more) for randomization, bootstrap, and Monte Carlo methods. Particularly useful are his chapters on time series data and spatial data. Time series data are often hard to analyze, and methods and examples are given for investigating hypotheses about serial correlation, trends, and periodicity. For spatial data, methods are given for investigating alternatives to random placement and also for determining whether two distance matrices are correlated. A simple example of a distance matrix is the one in a road atlas giving the distances between pairs of towns. Other types of distance (or similarity) matrix contain measures of how different or alike pairs of species, environments, or other items are (Dugard et al., 2010).

Randomization tests have been known for at least 70 years, but until fast, cheap computing was available to all researchers, most were not really usable. Efron remarked that an important theme for his work (1982) was the substitution of computational power for theoretical analysis. At an informal seminar the following year, he said that if we were to make as good use of the computational tools at our disposal as our forebears did of their primitive calculators, we would move statistics forward in great strides. Since then, there has been increasing interest in and development of randomization tests, and we hope this book will help to make them accessible to a wider audience.

Solutions to even numbered exercises

Chapter 2

2. A lot of computer power is needed to calculate the reference set, so not much progress was made with randomization tests until it was easily available.

4. There are 4!/(2!2!) or 24/4 or 6 ways to arrange 4 items, 2 each of 2 kinds. Here is a list.

   AABB ABAB BAAB BBAA BABA ABBA

6. The randomization method determines the reference set from which our actual experimental arrangement is taken. We have to compare our actual test statistic with the reference set, so we have to use the correct reference set.

8. If you just make one assignment at random and use it for all participants, you are choosing from only a few of the random assignments that are available for this experiment, and our macro assumes you choose from them all when calculating the reference set.

Chapter 3

2. If we have only one participant, or just a small group not chosen at random from a wider population, then we shall only learn whether our results apply more widely when further experiments are done with different participants. External validity accumulates gradually if similar results are found in different groups. When large-n designs are used, an essential feature is random assignment of participants to conditions, but participants are hardly ever chosen at random from the population to which we hope the results will apply. So even when a large-n design is used, external validity usually depends on repeating it in other centres or with different groups of patients.

4. If there may be some systematic variation from one day to the next, it may be better to treat each day as a block and assign the four conditions at random to observation periods within each day.

6. If we have only one participant, then we first have to decide whether the conditions to be investigated can be randomly assigned to observation occasions. Generally, this kind of random assignment is only possible for conditions where the effect only lasts while the condition is being applied. A good example would be pain killing drugs, but there are less obvious examples. For instance, different methods of behavior management in a classroom may only be effective while they are being actively applied. Among conditions which can't be applied at random to observation occasions are any with permanent or long lasting effects such as training or surgery. If conditions can be randomly applied to observation occasions then a one-way or repeated measures design may be considered. If random assignment is impossible or inappropriate, then a phase design may be the only option.

Chapter 4

2. The type of pain can't be randomly assigned to participant so pain type can't be a factor.

4. For each participant, the first possible intervention is point 4 and the last possible is point 8, giving 5 possibilities for each participant. Since 5*5 is 25, significance at 5% would be possible with just 2 participants.

6. Although the type of pain can't be a factor in a 2*2 factorial design, the type of pain could be a block. We could use a randomized blocks design with a block for each pain type. However, with 2 blocks and 2 conditions, there are only 2*2 or 4 possible arrangements. We really need a design where several participants use each type of pain reduction in each block. The macro for the small group repeated measures design with two conditions and replicates could be adapted like this. Let the pain type take the place of participants in the design as described in the chapter. So we will have 2 blocks (the pain types) and two conditions (the two kinds of pain reduction). The participants will be the replicates. Suppose for example that we have 6 willing participants in each pain category. So we have two blocks (pain types, like 2 participants in the chapter description), and we can take 6 measurements in each category (so the 6 participants are like the repeated measures). Assign the 6 participants in each block at random, 3 each to relaxation (R) and mindfulness (M) training. If there is no difference between the effects of R and M, then the labels are arbitrary and rearranging them within blocks will not change the

test statistic except by random variation. This is just what happens in the repeated measures with replicates macro: the condition labels are rearranged within participants. Within each pain type (block) there are 6!/(3!3!) or 20 possible arrangements of R, R, R, M, M and M. So we have 20*20 or 400 arrangements altogether, making significance at 5% a possibility even if we use a two-tailed test. Of course, it may be that R and M have different effects for the two kinds of pain, in which case we need to investigate them separately rather than average the effects across types of pain.

Chapter 5

2. The test statistic for the two-tailed test is just the test statistic for the one-tailed test but ignoring the sign (this is the absolute value). So if the test statistic for the one-tailed test is positive, its absolute value is just the same and the test statistic for the two-tailed test is just the same as that for the one-tailed test.

 Sometimes the one- and two-tailed probabilities are also the same, as we point out in the text. This result is likely with a phase design when the intervention has a large effect which is seen at every intervention observation.

4. Did you forget to edit the name ranges?

Chapter 6

2. There must be some randomization before a design can use the name. Conditions may be randomly assigned to participants or to observation occasions, or intervention and withdrawal points can be randomly assigned in phase designs.

4. Randomization enables us to secure internal validity.

6. Randomizing the intervention point for a phase design is the only way to achieve internal validity. Using response guided intervention maximizes the chance of finding a spurious effect.

8. Sometimes it may be worth doing the randomization test calculations even where there has been no randomization, perhaps as part of a preliminary investigation to decide whether to proceed with a line of enquiry. If this is done, then it must be made clear in reporting.

Chapter 7

2. If you find a probability close to 0.05 you may need a larger sample to get a better estimate. If you want to use the 1% significance level you probably need a sample of about 5000.

4. The power of the test is the probability of rejecting the null hypothesis when it is false, or the probability that you do not make a Type 2 error. The power of a test depends on the size. If you use a 1% significance level instead of 5% then you reduce the probability that the null hypothesis will be rejected, so you reduce the power. The power also depends on the effect size. You are more likely to reject the null hypothesis if there is a large effect than if the effect is small. Usually the power also depends on the number of participants or observations. Generally, larger n means higher power (but see the Onghena example in the text).

6. If we find an effect in rather artificial conditions, we may then pursue further knowledge of the circumstances where it is useful by investigating other groups of participants or other operating conditions. But if we miss an effect which is swamped by random variation then we may abandon a line of research which could have led to useful results.

8. Phase designs are quite unlikely to pick up clinically insignificant since their power is generally low unless effects are large.

Appendix 1: Basic skills for randomization tests

Choosing a random number within a given range

Do it with cards: the low-tech solution

Write each of the numbers from which we have to choose on a separate card (the cards should all be the same shape and size). Put the cards in a bag and shake it; then pull one out without looking into the bag. This is our chosen number.

Most calculators have a random number generator, so we could use that, but probably it will only give numbers between 0 and 1 so we need to do a bit of arithmetic to get a number in the range we want.

Use SPSS

Suppose we want to choose at random a number between 9 and 29 (perhaps for an intervention point in a phase design). In an empty datasheet, type a 1 at the top of the first column. Then from the menu choose **Transform** then **Compute Variable**. Scroll down the **Function group** list to **Random Numbers**, and select **Rv.Uniform**. Put it in the **Numeric expression** box by clicking the arrow. Now we need to replace the ?s in the brackets. Because SPSS will choose a number anywhere in the range we supply, not just whole numbers, we need to set the lowest value at a half below the smallest number in our range and set the highest value at a half above the highest in our range. This will ensure that the top and bottom numbers in our range have the same chance of being chosen as the ones in between. So to get a number between 9 and 29 as in our example, we need 8.5 and 29.5 as our values in the brackets. Give the random number a name in the **Target Variable** box, and click **OK** (see Figure A1.1 *SPSS Dialog Box A1.1*).

Return to the datasheet to find the chosen number at the top of column 2 (this would be our intervention point for the phase design). If decimal places

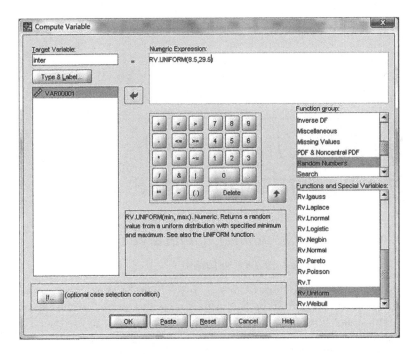

Figure A1.1 *SPSS Dialog Box A1.1* Choosing a random number between 9 and 29.

are shown, round to the closest whole number (or go to **Variable view** and reduce the decimal points displayed to zero so SPSS does this for you).

If we want several random numbers in the same range, put more numbers in column 1. For example, if we put numbers 1, 2, and 3 in the first three rows of column 1, then there will be three random numbers in our chosen range (from 9 to 29 in our example) in the first three rows of column 2.

Use Excel

Excel will pick a number between 9 and 29 at random if we enter **=randbetween(9,29)** in an empty cell. Because Excel chooses a whole number in the specified range, we don't need to take 8.5 as the lowest and 29.5 as the highest (like in SPSS) to give 9 and 29 the same chance of being chosen as the other numbers.

Arranging a set of objects in random order

To arrange objects in random order, we need to number them. For example suppose we have an experiment where we need to present to our participants 10 different symbols in random order. First we just number the symbols from 1 to 10.

The objects to be arranged in random order need not all be different. For instance, if want to arrange treatments randomly over observation occasions, we will have several occasions for each treatment. Suppose we have three treatments and eight observation occasions. Treatments 1 and 2 are to get three occasions each, and treatment 3 is to get two occasions. So we want to arrange 1, 1, 1, 2, 2, 2, 3, and 3 in random order. The methods described below work equally well for objects that are all different or objects that have several copies of each type. It is also possible to arrange symbols in random order using the same methods. For instance we could arrange the four Vs and four Ns from the ESP experiment in random order.

Do it with cards: the low-tech solution

Write the numbers (or symbols) on separate cards, put them in a bag, shake it up, and pull them out one at a time to give you a random order for the objects. If we are randomly ordering the 10 symbols from our example and the symbols are already printed on separate equally sized cards, we can just put these cards in the bag, shake it, and pull them out one at a time. We can actually do this at the time of the experiment if we wish, but we may still want to record the order in which the symbols were presented. For the example of three treatments above, we need eight cards with the numbers 1, 1, 1, 2, 2, 2, 3, and 3. For the ESP experiment we would need eight cards, four with a V and four with an N.

Use SPSS

We can get a random ordering of any set of numbers from SPSS as follows. To be definite we will use the numbers 1 to 10, but our numbers need not all be different. We could also use letters, for example V, V, V, V, N, N, N, and N for the ESP experiment. For the example using numbers 1 to 10, create a column of numbers 1 to 10 (we called it x in Figure A1.2 *SPSS Dialog Box A1.2*). In **Variable view**, reduce the number of decimal places displayed for x to zero. Then from the menu choose **Transform**, then **Compute Variable**. Select **Random numbers** in the **Function group** box, and put **Rv.Uniform** from the **Functions and Special variables** box into the **Numeric Expression** box with the arrow (see Figure A1.1 *SPSS Dialog Box A1.1*). Replace the first **?** with 0 for the lowest value and the second **?** with 1 for the highest value. Give a name to the **Target Variable** (RANDOM would do). Click **OK** and we will have 10 numbers between 0 and 1 in a new column called RANDOM. Now from the menu choose **Data**, then **Sort Cases** and put RANDOM in the **Sort by** box with the arrow. Click **OK**. This will sort the rows into order according to the values in the RANDOM column. The column called x now contains the numbers 1 to 10 in random

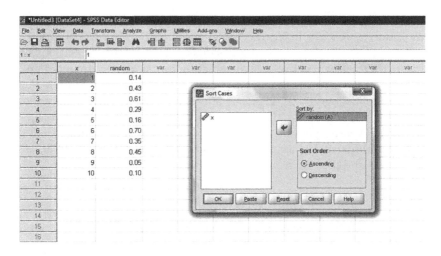

Figure A1.2 SPSS Dialog Box A1.2 Obtaining a random ordering of numbers 1 to 10.

order. We have just used the numbers 1 to 10 to illustrate the process, but we can put any set of numbers for which we want a random ordering in the x column. The set of numbers does not have to start with 1 and the numbers need not be all different. We could use 1, 1, 1, 2, 2, 2, 3, and 3 from the treatment example above to get a random order of treatments over observation occasions. We could also put V, V, V, V, N, N, N, and N in the column called x, make a column of random numbers and sort as described above, to get the V and N sessions in random order for the ESP experiment.

Use Excel

In column A put the numbers we want arranged in random order. To be definite we will arrange the numbers 1 to 10 in random order, but our numbers need not all be different and need not begin with 1. Now in cell B1 create a random number using =RAND(), and copy this down through cells B2 to B10. We now have 10 random numbers between 0 and 1 in cells B1 to B10. Select columns A and B, then click the **Data** tab on the menu bar. Open the **Sort** dialog box by clicking the **Sort** icon in the **Sort and Filter** group. Put column B in the **Sort by** box as shown in Figure A1.3 *Excel Datasheet A1.1*, and click **OK**.

The numbers in column A will be arranged in random order. If we have the treatment numbers 1, 1, 1, 2, 2, 2, 3, and 3 in column A, then we should only copy the formula from B1 into cells B2 to B8 because there are only 8 numbers. In general, copy the =RAND() formula so that column B is the same length as column A. To arrange four Vs and four Ns in random

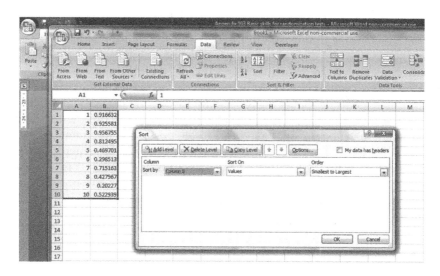

Figure A1.3 *Excel Datasheet A1.1* Obtaining a random ordering of numbers 1 to 10.

order for the ESP experiment, just put V, V, V, V, N, N, N, and N in column A and random numbers in B1 to B8 as before. Sort on column B exactly as before to get a random ordering of the four Vs and four Ns.

Listing and counting intervention points for phase designs

The single-case AB design

For this design, once we know how many observations we can make, and the minimum number in each phase, it is straightforward to list the possible intervention points. To be definite, suppose we can make 25 observations and we need at least 6 for the baseline and at least 8 for the intervention phase. So the first observation we could make for the intervention phase would be number 7 (leaving the first 6 for the baseline). We could also intervene at numbers 8, 9, 10, 11, and so on up to number 18. But we couldn't intervene as late as number 19 because that would only leave 7 observations (19, 20, 21, 22, 23, 24, and 25) for the intervention phase, and we need 8. So we have 12 possible intervention points (25 − 6 − 8 + 1).

The AB multiple baseline design

Here we suppose we have several participants and we will choose the intervention point at random separately for each one. Suppose we have 2 participants and we make 25 observations on each, with at least 6 in the baseline phase and at least 8 in the intervention phase. Then, as we saw for the single-case above, the first possible intervention point for participant 1 is point 7 and the last is 18, giving 12 possible intervention points. Once an intervention point in the range 7–18 is chosen at random for the first participant, we repeat the process for the second participant. Because any of the 12 possible points for participant 1 can be paired with any of the 12 for participant 2, we have 12*12 or 144 possible arrangements. If we have more participants, to calculate the number of arrangements for the experiment, multiply 12 by itself the same number of times as we have participants. For a different number of possible intervention points for each participant, replace 12 by the new number of possible intervention points.

The single-case ABA design

Here we need to know the total number of observations and the minimum number needed in each of the three phases (baseline, intervention, and withdrawal). To be definite, suppose we can make 14 observations and we need at least three in each phase. So the first point where we could have the intervention would be observation 4, leaving observations 1, 2, and 3 for the baseline. If the intervention starts at point 4, the first point at which we could start withdrawal would be point 7, leaving 4, 5, and 6 for the intervention. This would leave 8 observations for the withdrawal phase (points 7, 8, 9, 10, 11, 12, 13, and 14). But we could also start the withdrawal at points 8, 9, 10, 11, or 12. Any later and we won't have at least 3 points left for the withdrawal phase. Now suppose the intervention starts at point 5. Withdrawal then can't begin until at least point 8 (leaving 5, 6, and 7 for the intervention phase). But we could also have the withdrawal at points 9, 10, 11, or 12. The latest we could start the intervention and still leave at least 3 points each for the intervention and withdrawal phases would be point 9 (9, 10, and 11 for the intervention phase, 12, 13, and 14 for withdrawal). The list of possible pairs looks like this.

(4,7) (4,8) (4,9) (4,10) (4,11) (4,12)
    (5,8) (5,9) (5,10) (5,11) (5,12)
        (6,9) (6,10) (6,11) (6,12)
           (7,10) (7,11) (7,12)
              (8,11) (8,12)
                (9,12)

So there are 21 pairs. To choose a pair for our study, number the pairs in our list and then choose a random number between 1 and the number of pairs in the list (21 here). The pair that corresponds to our random number is the one to use.

The ABA multiple baseline design

Just as in the multiple baseline AB design, any intervention pair for participant 1 can be combined with any pair from subject 2, so if we have just 2 subjects and the same constraints as for the single-case ABA design above we would have 21*21 or 441 possible choices. Choose the pair of points for participant 1 from the list above, then choose again for participant 2, and again until we have chosen for every participant.

Checking for serial correlation

To check to see if neighboring values are correlated in case, for example, one score influences the next, we need to correlate the data with the same data shifted down one row or more rows.

In the SPSS datasheet, if the observations to be checked for serial correlation form a variable (column), just copy the variable into a new column, but one row lower down. From the menu bar choose **Analyze**, then **Correlate** and **Bivariate**. Put the original variable and the one we made by copying, into the **Variables** box using the arrow, and click **OK**. The datasheet with 20 example observations and the dialog box is shown as Figure A1.4 *SPSS Dialog Box A1.3*. The correlation is 0.026.

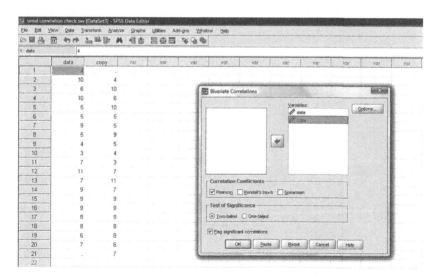

Figure A1.4 *SPSS Dialog Box A1.3* Checking for serial correlation.

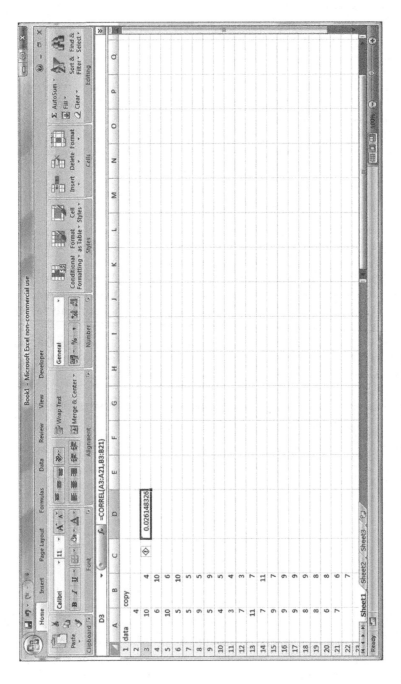

Figure A1.5 Excel Datasheet A1.2 Checking for serial correlation.

In Excel, use the **CORREL** function from the list of statistical functions. Enter as **Array 1** our observations from point 2 (row 3) to the end and enter as **Array 2** our copy from point 1 (row 3) to the penultimate point (row 21). This is shown in Figure A1.5 *Excel Datasheet A1.2.*

The correlation between neighboring values is called the *lag 1 correlation*: it is the correlation of each observation with the one that follows it. To get the *lag 2 correlation*, copy the original variable into a new column but two rows lower.

Appendix 2: SPSS macros

Introduction

The first section of this appendix, "Running a Macro in SPSS," should be useful to anyone wanting to use our macros to analyze their data. The remainder of this appendix, starting with the section "Editing a Macro in SPSS," is needed only if you want to understand the macros to modify them or write your own. If you just want to use our macros as they are, you can skip these later sections.

Running a macro in SPSS

The first step in using our macros is to go to the book Web site (http://www.researchmethodsarena.com/9780415886932) and download both the macro syntax files (with extension *.sps*) and the example data files (with extension *.sav*), and save them in a suitable place on your own computer. After trying out the macros with the example data, edit the data files to replace the example data with your own, but retain the names for the variables. We will demonstrate running an SPSS macro using that for the one-way design with the single-case example data.

First make sure you have the data in the active datasheet. Use **File > Open > Data** and browse to find the correct data file (*onewaysinglecase.sav*) if it's not already open. Then you need to open the syntax file that contains the macro. This time use **File > Open > Syntax** and browse to find and open the file *oneway.sps*. The macro appears in the syntax window as shown in Figure A2.1 *SPSS Syntax A2.1*. Now select **Run** on the menu bar as shown, and click **All** to run the macro.

In a few moments, the results appear in the output window as shown in Figure A2.2 *SPSS Output A2.1*. Note that the results will not be exactly the same as ours because a different random sample is used for each run.

You can run the macro again by returning to the syntax window (use **Window** on the menu bar) and use **Run** and then **All** again.

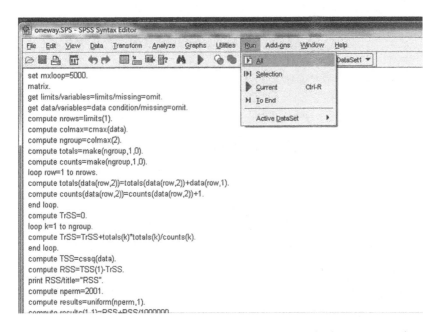

Figure A2.1 *SPSS Syntax A2.1* The one-way macro appearing in the syntax window.

```
Run MATRIX procedure:

RSS
    4.666666667

count of arrangement RSS at least as small
    742

probability
    .3713143428

------ END MATRIX -----
```

Figure A2.2 *SPSS Output A2.1.*

Editing a macro in SPSS

The remainder of this appendix need be read only by those wishing to adapt our macros or write their own. If you are writing your own, you should also consult Chapter 8.

The easiest way to edit a macro is to open it in the syntax window (using **File > Open > Syntax**) and make the changes you want. It's a useful precaution to make a copy of the original and give it a new name such as "temp" while you try out alterations. You can do this using **File > Save As** and entering "temp" in the File Name box. The name at the top of the window changes to temp.sps, and you can try ideas out. The original macro is still stored under the original name. Once you are satisfied with your edits, of course give your new macro a sensible name that will help you to locate it when needed.

You can try out alterations as soon as you make them by using **Run > All**, as long as you have suitable data in the active datasheet. Often you need several attempts to get a change working correctly. While you work on it, you may want to reduce the size of the reference set sample to something quite small, perhaps 10 or 20. If you want to try out just a few lines, you can select them and then **Run > Selection**. If you can't get the macro to do what you want, it may help in working out what the problem is if you write in extra lines to give intermediate steps in a calculation. For example, you could insert

```
print data.
```

after the loop where you rearrange the data, so you can see whether your efforts to rearrange the data in the way required by the design are working properly. You can easily remove any extra commands, and put the size of the reference set back up if you reduced it, once you have it working properly.

Writing a macro in SPSS

You can write a macro in the syntax window and try it out a bit at a time as explained in the "Editing a Macro in SPSS" section. But perhaps the most likely thing for you to want to do yourself is to use or adapt parts of our macros to analyze designs for which we have not provided a macro. A first step for this task would be understanding the macros we have provided, and to this end we offer listings of all our macros, general notes in the "Understanding the Macros" section, and additional notes with each macro. In the general notes we explain a few of the techniques that are used in nearly every macro. As we go through the macro listings, we give an explanation of each technique when it is used for the first time. If the same technique is used in a later macro, we only sketch the explanation and refer you back to its first appearance. In addition, Chapter 8 includes a section where we document the process of using and adapting part of one of the macros in order to produce a new one for a new design. We offer this example to show you the process in action. We should warn you that gaining the understanding you need to produce macros on your own is hard work. Often you need to work through a group of lines using example numbers to see how they work, especially as you try to understand how we do the rearrangements.

Understanding the macros

In this section, we list the syntax for the SPSS macros with added notes. We begin with a few general notes that apply to nearly every macro, and then proceed to the annotated listings.

Introduction and general notes

All the macros follow this pattern.

1. Begin by increasing the number of iterations SPSS will do.
2. Set up two matrices to hold the number of observations, the observations, and the condition codes.
3. Find the test statistic for the actual experiment.
4. The main part of the macro performs the rearrangements and calculates the rearrangement test statistics to form the reference set.
5. Compare values in the reference set with the actual test statistic.
6. Finally, two-tailed (and one-tailed, where appropriate) test probabilities are calculated and printed.

1. Begin by increasing the number of iterations SPSS will do

All the macros use loops get the 2000 random samples from the reference set. There is a default maximum number allowed by SPSS that is less than this, so we always begin by increasing to 5000, which will still do if you decide on a larger random sample from the reference set. Here's the command.

```
set mxloop=5000.
```

2. Set up two matrices to hold the number of observations, the observations, and the condition codes

The macros use the SPSS matrix language, and if you want to write your own or make more than trivial adaptations to ours, you will need to learn a bit about it. The most important thing is that a matrix is just a set of columns, where each element can be identified by its row and column. The matrix language is started by the command "matrix." and ended with the command "end matrix." Note that all commands end in a full stop.

The macros usually begin by setting up two matrices, one called LIM-ITS with only one column to contain information about numbers of observations and sometimes other details of the experiment, and another called DATA with several columns to contain the observations and codes for conditions, factor levels or participants. For the one-way design, (single-case example data in Table 4.1), the LIMITS matrix contains only one number, 9, which is the number of observations in the first column of the datasheet. The DATA matrix for this design has two columns: The first is the second column of the datasheet (the one called DATA), and the second is the third column of the datasheet (called CONDITION). So, for example, the fourth row, second column of the DATA matrix is number 2; and the fifth row, first column is number 4. Here are the commands for the one-way design, and there are similar ones near the beginning of every macro.

```
get limits/variables=limits/missing=omit.
get data/variables=data condition/missing=omit.
```

Cases with missing values will be omitted. Notice that the second command, to set up the DATA matrix, uses the column names (DATA and CONDITION) from the datasheet that contains the observations and the condition codes. As you will see in some of the later macros, there may be more than two columns in the DATA matrix. For example, the two-way factorial design has three columns called DATA, FACTOR1, and FACTOR2 in the datasheet (Table 4.8), and these become three columns in the DATA matrix.

3. Find the test statistic for the actual experiment

We often have to accumulate totals of observations for each condition or factor level. This is usually achieved by keeping a running total using a loop that starts the total at zero and then steps through the observations, adding each one to the correct total for its condition or factor level. We need to start this process with totals that are zero; we need a zero total for each condition or factor level. For the one-way design (Table 4.1), we have three conditions, so we need three totals. In each macro, we either have to put the number of conditions in the LIMITS column or else get the macro to work it out in some way. In the one-way design, it is the highest number in column 2 of the data matrix (the condition codes). Here are the commands.

```
compute colmax=cmax(data).
compute ngroup=colmax(2).
```

So, for this example, ngroup will be 3, the highest condition code, and this is the number of conditions.

Now we set up a column of zero totals (there are three for our current example). So we start with a matrix called TOTALS with three rows (in this example), one column, and all entries zero.

```
compute totals=make(ngroup,1,0).
```

If the design always has only two conditions (as in the one-way design with two conditions, for instance), you may need only two totals to start at zero, and then you may see a command like this instead:

```
compute totals={0,0}.
```

Now we need to step through each observation (one in each row) with a loop. The number of rows has to be read from the LIMITS column or else calculated from other values in the LIMITS column. For the one-way design, the number of rows of data is just the single number in the LIMITS column. Here's the command (the number of rows is 9 for the current example).

```
compute nrows=limits(1).
```

So the loop will be started with the command

```
loop row=1 to nrows.
```

and ended with the command

```
end loop.
```

To do the step-by-step additions, we have to add each observation to the correct total. As we loop through, we first need to decide which total to use by finding out in which condition the observation was made. For a particular observation, say the third (row = 3), the correct total is found by looking in row 3 and column 2 of the matrix called DATA, which contains the condition code for the third observation. This will be the number in DATA(3,2). In general, we find the condition code for the row we are on by looking at in DATA(row,2). The observation for the row we are on will be in DATA(row,1). So the matrix language does the additions in a very concise way. We add DATA(row,1) to the DATA(row,2) row of the TOTALS matrix using this command.

```
totals(data(row,2))=totals(data(row,2))+data(row,1).
```

Using the data in Table 4.1, the observation in the third row is 2 and it was obtained in condition 1. So for the third step in the process, the command says,

```
compute totals(1) = totals(1) + 2
```

Sometimes we use a similar method for counting the number of observations in a condition, as here:

```
compute counts(data(row,2))=counts(data(row,2))+1.
```

Once again the condition code for the current step (row = 3 to continue our previous example) is found in column 2 of the DATA matrix. But we are counting, not totaling, so we add only 1 to the appropriate count.

The test statistic is not the same for all macros, and you will see the specific commands needed as you work through the macros, but some variation on the steps just described is used in all macros.

4. The main part of the macro performs the rearrangements and calculates the rearrangement test statistics to form the reference set

We have to set the size of the random sample from the reference set. We always use 2000, but it's easy to change. The command is this one:

```
compute nperm=2001.
```

The number is 2001 because the first value is the one from the actual experiment, then we do 2000 rearrangements for the random sample from the reference set.

Further into the macro, we have to define matrices to hold the reference set and sometimes also intermediate calculations on the way to getting the reference set. To define a matrix, you have to put something in it, and we have often used the device of filling up a matrix with uniform random numbers. It really doesn't matter what goes in; you just need a quick way to do it, then as the values you need are calculated, they replace the numbers you used to set up the matrix. So in most macros you see this command (remember nperm was set to 2001).

```
compute results=uniform(nperm,1).
```

This makes a matrix with one column, and the number of rows is 1 plus the number of random samples we take from the reference set (usually 2001, including the one from the actual experiment).

Rearrangements are obtained using random numbers. Uniform(1,1) is a random number between 0 and 1, where the probability is spread evenly along the interval from 0 to 1. The probability of exactly 0 or exactly 1 is vanishingly small and can be ignored. Often we multiply uniform(1,1) by some whole number and then *truncate* the answer to get a random number in the range we want. For instance, 5*uniform(1,1) gives a random number between 0 and 5 (with exactly 0 or 5 being vanishingly improbable), so truncating it gives a whole number between 0 and 4.

We store the test statistic from the actual experiment in the first position in the RESULTS matrix, RESULTS(1,1), the first place in the first and only column. The test statistics from the rearrangements, our random sample from the reference set, occupy the other 2000 places in the column and are put in as we calculate them. The actual test statistic has to be compared with the ones calculated from the 2000 rearrangements, and we need to count how many are larger (or sometimes smaller) than our actual one from the experiment. We found that SPSS sometimes was unable to decide the result of comparing two numbers that are equal. To deal with this, we reduced the actual test statistic by a very small multiple of itself so it could always be compared even if a reference set value was the same. The effect will be to make the test marginally more *conservative*. (If we are looking to see if our test statistic is smaller than those in the reference set, we increase it by a very small multiple of itself, which again makes the test marginally more conservative.) Here is an example from the one-way design, where the test statistic is the residual sum of squares (RSS), so we shall be interested in whether it is smaller than the majority of the reference set.

```
compute results(1,1)=RSS+RSS/1000000.
```

5. Compare values in the reference set with the actual test statistic
The comparisons and count are achieved by stepping through the reference set from numbers 2 to 2001, adding to the count if the reference set value is at least as large as (or sometimes at least as small as) the actual test statistic. Here the count is called pos, and we started it from zero in an earlier command. If one- and two-tailed tests are both available, we need pos1 and pos2. Here is the comparison and counting process for the RSS example used above:

```
loop k=2 to nperm.
do if results(k,1)<=results(1,1).
compute pos=pos+1.
end if.
end loop.
```

6. Finally two-tailed (and one-tailed, where appropriate) test probabilities are calculated and printed
The final step in all macros is achieved with some commands like these, where we print titles, the pos count, and the probability (here just the two-

tailed). To get the probability, we need the count of values from the reference set to be at least as extreme as the actual test statistic, plus 1 for the experimental one (pos+1). Then divide by the number of values from the reference set plus 1 for the experimental value (nperm, or 2001 in this example).

```
print pos/title="count of arrangement RSS at least as small".
compute prob=(pos+1)/nperm.
print prob/title="probability".
```

There is more than you need to know about all this in the SPSS **Help** file (go to **Topics** and type **matrix language** in the search box). Now we list each macro with some further comments in bold. Please note that where the page width prevents us getting a complete command on one line, we use *c* as our continuation symbol. There is always room for the full command in the SPSS syntax window, so omit the *c* if typing such a line yourself.

For the first macro, we include the step numbers (but not the headings) from the previous section.

One-way design (single-case or small-n)

The required files are *oneway.sps* (syntax for the macro) and *onewaysinglecase.sav* (single-case example data) or *onewaysmallgroup.sav* (small-*n* example data).

You can look at the example data in Tables 4.1 and 4.2. We quote values from Table 4.1 in the explanations for this macro.

1 and 2. Increase the maximum loop size, start the matrix language, and make two matrices: LIMITS, which just contains the total number of observations, and DATA containing the observations (column 1) and condition codes (column 2).

```
set mxloop=5000.          increase the maximum loop size to 5000
matrix.                   start the matrix language
get limits/variables=limits/missing=omit.
                          form a matrix from the first column of the
                          data window
get data/variables=data condition/missing=omit.
                          form a matrix from the second and third
                          columns of the data window
```

3. Now use the information from the datasheet stored in LIMITS to set the number of observations (nrows) and the number of conditions (ngroup).

To find the number of conditions, we need the highest condition code, so use the column maximum function, cmax, to get the maximum for both columns of the DATA matrix, then take the maximum from column 2 as the number of conditions.

```
compute nrows=limits(1).      find the number of rows of data from the
                              top of the LIMITS column (9 in the
                              example)
compute colmax=cmax(data).    find the highest number in each column
                              of DATA (in the example, 4 for column 1
                              and 3 for column 2)
compute ngroup=colmax(2).     the number of conditions is the highest
                              number in column 2 (3 in the example)
```

Now we start the job of calculating the actual test statistic from the experiment. We are going to use the RSS, so we need condition (treatment or group) totals and counts from which to get treatment sum of squares.

```
compute totals=make(ngroup,1,0).   make a matrix of zeros with ngroup
                                   rows, one for each condition (3 in
                                   the example), and one column to
                                   receive the condition totals
compute counts=make(ngroup,1,0).   and another for the counts
```

To find the totals and counts for the actual experiment, step through the data assigning each observation the correct total as described in the introduction to this section.

```
loop row=1 to nrows.               nrows is 9 for the example, so 9
                                   steps in the loop
compute totals(data(row,2))=totals(data(row,2))+data(row,1).
                                   this key step is explained in the
                                   introductory section
compute counts(data(row,2))=counts(data(row,2))+1.
end loop.
```

Here the test statistic is the residual sum of squares. To get the RSS, we need the condition (treatment or group) SS for each condition (called TrSS), just like in ANOVA. We also need the total SS (TSS), and the function cssq finds the SS for each column of data. We just use that from the first column, which contains the observations.

```
compute TrSS=0.              collect the condition SS for the actual
                             data, starting with zero
loop k=1 to ngroup.          and adding in the contribution from each
                             condition
compute TrSS=TrSS+totals(k)*totals(k)/counts(k).
end loop.                    move to the next condition
compute TSS=cssq(data).      find the total SS for each column of DATA
compute RSS=TSS(1)-TrSS.     and the RSS which is the total SS from
                             the first column minus the condition SS
print RSS/title="RSS".       and print the answer
```

4. Now we start the job of getting the 2000 random samples from the reference set. We need to set the sample size (2000 plus one for the actual result from the experiment). Set up a matrix to contain the actual result at the top and the 2000 reference set values in positions 2 to 2001, and put the result for the actual experiment in the first place in the RESULTS matrix. As explained in the introduction, we increase our actual test statistic by a tiny amount to avoid comparison problems. Start the count of reference set values at least as small as our actual result at zero (pos = 0).

```
compute nperm=2001.                 set the number of samples
compute results=uniform(nperm,1).   make the results matrix
compute results(1,1)=RSS+RSS/1000000.  adjust the actual observation
                                    that is held in the first row
                                    of the results column as
                                    explained in the introductory
                                    section
compute pos=0.                      set to zero the starting
                                    value of the running count of
                                    examples more extreme than
                                    the observed one
```

Now we do 2000 rearrangements which will be numbers 2 to 2001 in the list of results.

```
loop perm=2 to nperm.               start the rearrangements
```

We can rearrange the condition codes while keeping the observations in place, or we can rearrange the observations while keeping the condition codes in place. It doesn't matter which we do, and we rearrange the observations, which are in column 1 of DATA.

We use uniform random numbers between 0 and 1, and to get a random number in the range we want, we multiply it by a whole number and then use just the integer part (truncate it with the function trunc).

We take the observations in turn (1 to nrows). At the first step, trunc(uniform(1,1)*(nrows-row+1) gives us a random number between 0 and nrows-1. Adding row (row = 1 at the first step) gives us a random number k between 1 and nrows. (Look again at the introduction and general notes for step 4.)

We put the first observation into a temporary store (temp = data(1,1)). Put the kth observation into data(1,1) and the first observation from temp into data(k,1).

At the next step, (row = 2) trunc(uniform(1,1)*(nrows-row+1) will be a random number between 0 and nrows-2, so k will be a random number between 2 and nrows. So at this step, we swap observation 2 with an observation between number 2 and nrows.

At any step, the swap may leave the observation in its original place. We continue the swapping process right down the list of observations, so at the end we have a rearrangement of the observations in the first column of DATA.

```
loop row=1 to nrows.                   nrows is 9 in the example
compute k=trunc(uniform(1,1)*(nrows-row+1))+row.
compute temp=data(row,1).
compute data(row,1)=data(k,1).
compute data(k,1)=temp.
end loop.
```

Once we have a rearrangement of the observations, we repeat the process above where we find the RSS, first getting the condition (treatment or group) totals and counts. We can reuse our totals and counts matrices by multiplying by zero to start them off at zero.

```
compute totals=0*totals.
compute counts=0*counts.
loop row=1 to nrows.
compute totals(data(row,2))=totals(data(row,2))+data(row,1).
compute counts(data(row,2))=counts(data(row,2))+1.
end loop.
```

Now get the test statistic RSS just as we did for the actual experiment, but using the totals and counts for the current arrangement. Put this RSS in the next place in the RESULTS matrix.

```
compute TrSS=0.
loop k=1 to ngroup.
compute TrSS=TrSS+totals(k)*totals(k)/counts(k).
end loop.
compute TSS=cssq(data).
compute RSS=TSS(1)-TrSS.
compute results(perm,1)=RSS.    put the RSS in the results matrix
end loop.                       now go to the next arrangement
```

5. Once we have 2000 values from the reference set, compare each with the actual RSS from the experiment. We are counting those at least as small.

```
loop k=2 to nperm.
do if results(k,1)<=results(1,1).
compute pos=pos+1.
end if.
end loop.
```

6. Now all we have to do is print the count of reference set values at least as small as the actual RSS from the experiment, and calculate the probability and print it.

```
print pos/title="count of arrangement RSS at least as small".
                               print the count
compute prob=(pos+1)/nperm.    calculate the probability
print prob/title="probability". and print it
end matrix.                     end of matrix language
```

One-way design (single-case or small-n) with just two conditions

The required files are *onewaytwoconditions.sps* (syntax for the macro) and *onewaytwoconditions.sav* (small-*n* example data). If a directional alternative hypothesis and a one-tailed test are to be used, the condition coded 2 must the one where the mean is predicted to be higher. The example data can be seen in Table 4.3.

The first part of this macro is just the same as for the one-way design above, except that as we have only two conditions, we don't need to get number of conditions (treatments or groups) from the column of condition codes and the TOTALS and COUNTS matrices have only two elements.

```
set mxloop 5000.        increase the maximum loop size to 5000
matrix.                 start the matrix language
```

```
get limits/variables=limits/missing=omit.
                            form a matrix from the first column of
                            the data window
get data/variables=data condition/missing=omit.
                            form a matrix from the second and third
                            columns of the data window
compute nrows =limits(1).    find the number of rows of data
compute totals={0;0}.        start the two condition totals and
compute counts={0;0}.        counts at zero
loop row =1 to nrows.        find the totals and counts for conditions
                            for the actual data
compute totals(data(row,2))=totals(data(row,2))+data(row,1).
compute counts(data(row,2))=counts(data(row,2))+1.
end loop.
```

Because we have only two conditions, we use the difference between condition means as the test statistic. We get both means in one step (the matrix language is very concise), but then we have to identify them by their row and column numbers (there's only one column) to get the test statistic.

```
compute means=totals/counts.          get the means
compute test=means(2,1)-means(1,1).   and the test statistic
print test/title="test statistic".    and print it
```

Just as in the previous macro, we set the sample size, and set up a matrix to contain the actual result at the top and the 2000 reference set values in positions 2 to 2001. We start the count of reference set values at least as large as our actual result at zero (pos1 = 0) for the one-tailed test. We also start a count at zero for the two-tailed test (pos2 = 0). This time we look for reference set values at least as large as our actual one from the experiment, so the actual test statistic is reduced by a small multiple of itself to avoid comparison problems.

```
compute nperm=2001.
compute results=uniform(nperm,1).
compute results(1,1)=test-test/1000000.
compute pos1=0.
compute pos2=0.
```

Now we do the rearrangements using exactly the same method as in the previous macro.

```
loop perm=2 to nperm
loop row=1 to nrows.
compute k=trunc(uniform(1,1)*(nrows-row+1))+row.
```

```
compute temp=data(row,1).
compute data(row,1)=data(k,1).
compute data(k,1)=temp.
end loop.
```

Once we have a rearrangement, we collect the condition totals and counts as before.

```
compute totals={0;0}.            start condition totals
compute counts={0;0}.            and counts at zero
loop row =1 to nrows.            collect totals and counts for
                                 conditions for this arrangement
compute totals(data(row,2))=totals(data(row,2))+data(row,1).
compute counts(data(row,2))=counts(data(row,2))+1.
end loop.
```

Calculate the condition means and the test statistic for this rearrangement just as we did for the actual data, and put it into the results matrix.

```
compute means=totals/counts.       find the means
compute test=means(2,1)-means(1,1).  and the test statistic
compute results(perm,1)=test.      and put in the results matrix
end loop.                          now go to the next arrangement
```

For the one-tailed test, we count the values from the reference set at least as large as our actual one, but for the two-tailed test we ignore the signs of values in the reference set and also our actual test statistic from the experiment. The function abs takes the values ignoring the signs. The comparisons and counts are done in exactly the same way as in the previous macro.

```
compute absres=abs(results).       find absolute values for two-
                                   tailed test
loop k=2 to nperm.                 step down the reference set values
do if results(k,1)>=results(1,1).  compare reference set values with
compute pos1=pos1+1.               the actual one, and count those
                                   at least as large
end if.
do if absres(k,1)>=absres(1,1).    and repeat the process for
                                   absolute values to get the
compute pos2=pos2+1.               two-tailed test
end if.
end loop.
```

Now all we have to do is print the counts and calculate and print the probabilities.

```
print pos1/title="count of arrangement statistics at least *c*
as large".
compute prob1=(pos1+1)/nperm.   calculate the one-tailed probability
print prob1/title="one tail probability".
print pos2/title="count of arrangement statistics at least *c*
as large in abs value as abs(test)".
compute prob2=(pos2+1)/nperm.   and the two-tailed probability
print prob2/title="two tail probability".
end matrix.                     end of the matrix language
```

A randomized blocks design (single-case or small-n repeated measures)

The required files are *randomizedblocks.sps* (syntax for the macro) and *randomizedblocks.sav* (single-case example data) or *repeatedmeasures.sav* (small-*n* repeated measures example). The example data can be seen in Tables 4.4 and 4.5.

We start off in the usual way, but notice that the data matrix has three columns this time.

```
set mxloops 5000.
matrix.
get limits/variables=limits/missing=omit.
get data/variables data condition block/missing omit.
```

From the LIMITS matrix, we find the number of rows of data. The number of conditions is the highest number in column 2 of the DATA matrix, and the number of blocks is the highest number in column 3 of DATA. We obtain these highest numbers with the function cmax, as we did in the one-way design.

```
compute nrows=limits(1).    collect the number of rows of data
compute colmax=cmax(data).  find the column maxima
compute nblock=colmax(3).   find the number of blocks (or participants)
compute ntreat=colmax(2).   find the number of conditions (treatments)
```

As in the one-way design, we use the RSS as the test statistic, and we need condition (treatment) and block totals to obtain it. We do not need counts because the symmetry of the design gives us the numbers of observations in each condition and block. As in the one-way design, we start the totals at zero and step through the observations, adding each to the appropriate totals.

```
compute totalt=make(ntreat,1,0).
compute totalb=make(nblock,1,0).
loop row=1 to nrows.
compute totalt(data(row,2))=totalt(data(row,2))+data(row,1).
                              the condition code for the
                              observation is in column 2
compute totalb(data(row,3))=totalb(data(row,3))+data(row,1).
                              and the block code is in column 3
end loop.
```

Now to get the test statistic, we need the condition (treatment) SS and also the block SS. Each is started at zero, then we add the contribution from each condition or block.

```
compute TrSS=0.          collect the condition SS for the actual data
loop tr=1 to ntreat.
compute TrSS=TrSS+totalt(tr)*totalt(tr)/nblock.
end loop.
compute BSS=0.           collect the block SS for the actual data
loop bl=1 to nblock.
compute BSS=BSS+totalb(bl)*totalb(bl)/ntreat.
end loop.
```

We get the total SS using the cssq function as in the one-way design. To get the correction term for the RSS, we use the csum function, which sums each column of the matrix (we only need the first column sum, the total of the observations).

```
compute sum=csum(data).    sum all the colulmns of DATA
compute corr=sum(1)*sum(1)/nrows.
                           and get the correction term for the RSS
compute TSS=cssq(data).    and the total SS
compute RSS=TSS(1)-TrSS-BSS+corr.
print RSS/title="RSS".     and the residual SS
```

Just as in the macro for the one-way design, we set the sample size, set up a matrix to contain the actual result at the top and the 2000 reference set values in positions 2 to 2001, and start the count of reference set values at least as small as our actual result at zero (pos = 0).

```
compute nperm=2001.
compute results=uniform(nperm,1)
compute results(1,1)=RSS+RSS/1000000.
compute pos=0.
```

Now we have to rearrange our observations within blocks. We do it one block at a time. The method used is the same as for the one-way design, but now we have to add an extra term to our number k to place us in the current block. We also have to work out which observation we are on. Each condition appears once in each block, so if for example we have 4 conditions and 3 blocks, when we are in block 2 and have reached condition 3, we are on observation 3+(2–1)*4.

```
loop perm=2 to nperm.              this loop takes us through the 2000
                                   arrangements
loop bl = 1 to nblock.             this loop takes each block in turn
loop tr = 1 to ntreat.             this is the loop that does the
                                   rearrangement
compute k=trunc(uniform(1,1)*(ntreat-tr+1))+tr+ntreat*(bl-1).
compute row=tr+ntreat*(bl-1).      this is the observation we have
                                   reached
compute temp=data(row,1).
compute data(row,1)=data(k,1).
compute data(k,1)=temp.
end loop.                          now move to the next observation in
                                   the current block
end loop.                          now move to the next block
```

Just as in the one-way design, we can reuse our condition and block totals by multiplying by zero each time we start a calculation of condition and block totals for a new arrangement. The condition and block totals for this arrangement are accumulated in exactly the same way as for the actual data from the experiment.

```
compute totalt=0*totalt.
compute totalb=0*totalb.
loop row=1 to nrows.
compute totalt(data(row,2))=totalt(data(row,2))+data(row,1).
compute totalb(data(row,3))=totalb(data(row,3))+data(row,1).
end loop.
```

Using the condition and block totals for this arrangement, obtain the RSS in exactly the same way as we did for the actual data from the experiment. Put the RSS in the next place in the RESULTS matrix.

```
compute TrSS=0.
loop tr=1 to ntreat.
compute TrSS=TrSS+totalt(tr)*totalt(tr)/nblock.
end loop.
compute BSS=0.
loop bl=1 to nblock.
compute BSS=BSS+totalb(bl)*totalb(bl)/ntreat.
end loop.
compute sum=csum(data).
compute corr=sum(1)*sum(1)/nrows.
compute TSS=cssq(data).
compute RSS=TSS(1)-TrSS-BSS+corr.
compute results(perm,1)=RSS.
end loop.                          go to the next arrangement
```

Now we have to compare the 2000 reference set values in the results matrix with the actual one from our experiment. This is just as we did it in the one-way design.

```
loop k=2 to nperm.
do if results(k,1)<=results(1,1).
compute pos=pos+1.
end if.
end loop.
```

Finally print the count, calculate and print the probability, and end the matrix language.

```
print pos/title="count of RSS as least as small".
compute prob=(pos+1)/nperm.
print prob/title="probability".
end matrix.
```

A randomized blocks design with two conditions (single-case or small-n repeated measures)

The macro is *randomizedblockstwoconditions.sps*, and the example data (single-case) is *randomizedblockstwoconditions.sav*. You can see the example data in Table 4.6.

The macro starts in exactly the same way as the previous one, with three columns in the DATA matrix. We know there are two conditions, so the number of rows of data is twice the number of blocks (or participants). The number of blocks is the only value in LIMITS.

```
set mxloops 5000.
matrix.
get limits/variables=limits/missing=omit.
get data/variables data condition block/missing omit.
compute nrows=limits(1)*2.
compute nblock=limits(1).
```

Because there are only two conditions, we shall use the difference between condition means as the test statistic. Start the condition totals at zero, and collect the totals exactly as in the one-way design.

```
compute total={0,0}.
loop row=1 to nrows.
compute total(data(row,2))=total(data(row,2))+data(row,1).
end loop.
```

The number of observations in each condition is the same as the number of blocks. Find and print the test statistic for the actual experiment. Set the sample size for the reference set. Set up a matrix to receive the results in the usual way, and put the actual test statistic at the top.

```
compute test=(total(2)-total(1))/nblock.
print test/title="test statistic".
compute nperm=2001.
compute results=uniform(nperm,1).
compute results(1,1)=test-test/1000000.
```

Now we have to rearrange the observations within blocks. We do it in exactly the same way as in the randomized blocks design above, taking the blocks in turn.

```
loop perm=2 to nperm.
loop bl = 1 to nblock.        take the blocks in turn
loop tr = 1 to 2.             this loop does the rearrangement
compute k=trunc(uniform(1,1)*(2-tr+1))+tr+2*(bl-1).
compute row=tr+2*(bl-1).      this is the observation we have reached
compute temp=data(row,1).
compute data(row,1)=data(k,1).
compute data(k,1)=temp.
end loop.
end loop.                     now go to the next block
```

When we have a rearrangement, we calculate the test statistic for it in exactly the same way as we did for the actual data, and put it in the next place in the RESULTS matrix.

```
compute total={0,0}.
loop row=1 to nrows.
```

```
compute totalt(data(row,2))=totalt(data(row,2))+data(row,1).
compute totals(data(row,3))=totals(data(row,3))+data(row,1).
end loop.
compute test=(totalt(2)-totalt(1))/nblock.
compute results(perm,1)=test.
end loop.                        now go to the next arrangement
```

For the one-tailed test, we count the values from the reference set at least as large as our actual one, but for the two-tailed test we ignore the signs of values in the reference set and also our actual test statistic from the experiment. The function abs takes the values ignoring the signs. The comparisons and counts are done in exactly the same way as in the one-way design with two conditions.

```
compute absres=abs(results).
compute pos1=0.
compute pos2=0.
loop k=2 to nperm.
do if results(k,1)>=results(1,1).
compute pos1=pos1+1.
end if.
do if absres(k,1)>=absres(1,1).
compute pos2=pos2+1.
end if.
end loop.
```

Now we only have to print the counts, calculate and print the one- and two-tailed probabilities just as in the one-way design with two conditions.

```
print pos1/title="count of arrangement statistics at least *c*
as large".
compute prob1=(pos1+1)/nperm.
print prob1/title="one tail probability".
print pos2/title="count of arrangement statistics at least *c*
as large in abs value as abs(test)".
compute prob2=(pos2+1)/nperm.
print prob2/title="two tail probability".
end matrix.                      end of the matrix language
```

Small-n repeated measures design with replicates

The macro is *smallgrouprepeatedmeasureswithreps.sps,* and the example data are *smallgrouprepeatedmeasureswithreps.sav.* You can see the example data in Table 4.7.

The macro starts in exactly the same way as the previous one, with three columns in the DATA matrix. The number of participants (ncase) is first in the LIMITS column, and the number of observations per participant (nswaps) is next. The number of rows of data (nobs) is the number of participants times the number of observations per participant.

```
set mxloops 5000.
matrix.
get limits/variables=limits/missing=omit.
get data/variables data condition participant/missing omit.
compute ncase=limits(1).
compute nswaps=limits(2).
compute nobs=ncase*nswaps.
```

Because there are only two conditions, we shall use the difference between condition means as our test statistic. To obtain this we need the condition totals, which are obtained in exactly the same way as in the one-way design with two conditions. The number of observations per condition is half the number of observations, and this is what divides the difference between condition totals to get the test statistic.

```
compute total={0,0}.
loop obs=1 to nobs.
compute total(data(obs,2))=total(data(obs,2))+data(obs,1).
end loop.
compute test1=(total(2)-total(1))/(nobs/2).
print test1/title="test statistic".
```

Set the sample size for the reference set. Set up a matrix to receive the results in the usual way, and put the actual test statistic at the top.

```
compute nperm=2001.
compute results=uniform(nperm,1).
compute results(1,1)=test1-test1/1000000.
```

Now we have to rearrange the observations within participants, and we do it in the same way as we rearranged observations within blocks for the previous macro.

```
loop perm=2 to nperm.
loop case = 1 to ncase.    take the participants in turn
loop n= 1 to nswaps.       this is the loop that does the rearrangement
compute k=trunc(uniform(1,1)*(nswaps-n+1))+n+nswaps*(case-1).
compute obs=n+nswaps*(case-1).
compute temp=data(obs,1).
```

```
compute data(obs,1)=data(k,1).
compute data(k,1)=temp.
end loop.
end loop.                       now go to the next participant
```

When we have a rearrangement, we need to get the test statistic for it, and we do this in the same way as we obtained the test statistic for our actual experiment. Put the result in the next place in the RESULTS matrix.

```
compute total={0,0}.
loop obs=1 to nobs.
compute total(data(obs,2))=total(data(obs,2))+data(obs,1).
end loop.
compute test1=(total(2)-total(1))/(nobs/2).
compute results(perm,1)=test1.
end loop.                       now go to the next arrangement
```

For the one-tailed test, we count the values from the reference set at least as large as our actual one, but for the two-tailed test we ignore the signs of values in the reference set and also our actual test statistic from the experiment. The function abs takes the values ignoring the signs. The comparisons and counts are done in exactly the same way as in the one-way design with two conditions.

```
compute absres=abs(results).
compute pos1=0.
compute pos2=0.
loop k=2 to nperm.
do if results(k,1)>=results(1,1).
compute pos1=pos1+1.
end if.
do if absres(k,1)>=absres(1,1).
compute pos2=pos2+1.
end if.
end loop.
```

Now we only have to print the counts, calculate and print the one- and two-tailed probabilities just as in the one-way design with two conditions.

```
print pos1/title="count of arrangement statistics at least *c*
as large".
compute prob1=(pos1+1)/nperm.
print prob1/title="one tail probability".
print pos2/title="count of arrangement statistics at least *c*
as large in abs value as abs(test)".
```

```
compute prob2=(pos2+1)/nperm.
print prob2/title="two tail probability".
end matrix.
```

Two-way factorial design (single-case or small-n)

The required files are *factorial.sps* (syntax for the macro) and *factorial-singlecase.sav* (single-case example data) or *factorialsmallgroup.sav* (small-*n* example data). You can also look at the data in Tables 4.8 and 4.9.

This macro has separate parts for factor 1 and factor 2. The output appears separated by the parts of the macro listing. This device is necessary because the data have to be correctly ordered before each part, and sorting must be done outside the matrix language. If the data are presented as in Tables 4.8 and 4.9, the first sort shouldn't be necessary, but we include it as an extra check. Notes are provided only for the first part. In the second part, the two factors reverse roles.

As always, we increase the number of iterations SPSS will do. Then we sort the data into order by the levels of factor 2.

```
set mxloops 5000.          increase the maximum loop size to 5000
sort cases by factor2(A).  arrange the data according to levels of
                           factor 2 (A for ascending order)
```

Now we proceed as usual. Note that the DATA matrix contains three columns: observations (column 1), factor 1 levels (column 2), and factor 2 levels (column 3).

```
matrix.
get limits/variables=limits/missing=omit.
get data/variables data factor1 factor2/missing omit.
```

The total number of observations is all we need to find the number in each combination of factor levels (nreps) and the number at each level of factor 2 (nswaps) for rearranging within levels of factor 2.

```
compute nobs=limits(1).      total number of observations
compute nreps=limits(1)/4.   number of replicates
compute nswaps=limits(1)/2.  number of observations at each level of
                             factor 2
```

The factor 1 test statistic is the difference between level 2 and level 1 means, so we need observation totals for each level of factor 1. The matrix TOTALF1 will contain these totals. Start the totals at zero because they are accumulated by moving down the list of observations adding each to the appropriate total just as in the one-way design. Use the totals and the number of observations at each level of factor 1 to get the means and hence test statistic. Notice that the number of observations at each level of factor 1 is nobs/2 or nreps*2.

```
compute totalf1={0,0}.
loop obs=1 to nobs.
compute totalf1(data(obs,2))=totalf1(data(obs,2))+data(obs,1).
end loop.
compute test1=(totalf1(2)-totalf1(1))/(nreps*2).
print test1/title="factor 1 test statistic".
```

Set the sample size for the reference set. Set up a matrix to receive the results in the usual way, and put the actual test statistic at the top.

```
compute nperm=2001.
compute results1=uniform(nperm,1).
compute results1(1,1)=test1-test1/1000000.
```

We need to rearrange the observations within levels of factor 2, just as we rearranged observations within blocks for the randomized blocks design. The same method is used here. We take each level of factor 2 in turn, and rearrange observations within it.

```
loop perm=2 to nperm.
loop fac2 = 1 to 2.              take factor 2 levels in turn
loop n= 1 to nswaps.            this loop does the rearrangement
compute k=trunc(uniform(1,1)*(nswaps-n+1))+n+nswaps*(fac2-1).
compute obs=n+nswaps*(fac2-1).  this works out which observation we
                                have reached
compute temp=data(obs,1).
compute data(obs,1)=data(k,1).
compute data(k,1)=temp.
end loop.
end loop.                       now move to the next factor 2 level
```

When we have a rearrangement, we need to calculate the test statistic, and we do it in exactly the same way as we did for the actual experiment, starting the factor 1 level totals at zero and adding each observation to the appropriate total. When we have the test statistic, put it in the next place in the RESULTS1 matrix.

```
compute totalf1={0,0}.
loop obs=1 to nobs.
compute totalf1(data(obs,2))=totalf1(data(obs,2))+data(obs,1).
```

```
end loop.
compute test1=(totalf1(2)-totalf1(1))/(nreps*2).
compute results1(perm,1)=test1.
end loop.                                    move to the next arrangement
```

For the one-tailed test, we count the values from the reference set at least as large as our actual one, but for the two-tailed test we ignore the signs of values in the reference set and also our actual test statistic from the experiment. The function abs takes the values ignoring the signs. The comparisons and counts are done in exactly the same way as in the one-way design with two conditions.

```
compute absres1=abs(results1).
compute pos1=0.
compute pos2=0.
loop k=2 to nperm.
do if results1(k,1)>=results1(1,1).
compute pos1=pos1+1.
end if.
do if absres1(k,1)>=absres1(1,1).
compute pos2=pos2+1.
end if.
end loop.
```

Once the comparisons are done and values at least as large counted, we just have to calculate one- and two-tailed probabilities and print the results.

```
print pos1.
compute prob1=(pos1+1)/nperm.
print prob1/title=" factor 1 one tail probability".
print pos2.
compute prob2=(pos2+1)/nperm.
print prob2/title=" factor 1 two tail probability".
end matrix.                                  end of the matrix language
```

This is the end of Part 1. Part 2 can start as soon as we arrange the data in order by factor 1 levels.

```
sort cases by factor1(A).    arrange the data according to levels of
                             factor 1
matrix.                      restart the matrix language for part 2
get limits/variables=limits/missing=omit.
get data/variables data factor1 factor2/missing omit.
compute nobs=limits(1).
```

```
compute nreps=limits(1)/4.
compute nswaps=limits(1)/2.
compute results2=uniform(nperm,1).
compute totalf2={0,0}.
loop obs=1 to nobs.
compute totalf2(data(obs,3))=totalf2(data(obs,3))+data(obs,1).
end loop.
compute test2=(totalf2(2)-totalf2(1))/(nreps*2).
print test2/title="factor 2 test statistic".
compute nperm=2001.
compute results2=uniform(nperm,1).
compute results2(1,1)=test2-test2/1000000.
loop perm=2 to nperm.
loop fac1 = 1 to 2.
loop n= 1 to nswaps.
compute k=trunc(uniform(1,1)*(nswaps-n+1))+n+nswaps*(fac1-1).
compute obs=n+nswaps*(fac1-1).
compute temp=data(obs,1).
compute data(obs,1)=data(k,1).
compute data(k,1)=temp.
end loop.
end loop.
compute totalf2={0,0}.
loop obs=1 to nobs.
compute totalf2(data(obs,3))=totalf2(data(obs,3))+data(obs,1).
end loop.
compute test2=(totalf2(2)-totalf2(1))/(nreps*2).
compute results2(perm,1)=test2.
end loop.
compute absres2=abs(results2).
compute pos1=0.
compute pos2=0.
loop k=2 to nperm.
do if
results2(k,1)>=results2(1,1).
compute pos1=pos1+1.
end if.
do if
absres2(k,1)>=absres2(1,1).
compute pos2=pos2+1.
end if.
end loop.
print pos1.
compute prob1=(pos1+1)/nperm.
print prob1/title=" factor 2 one tail probability".
```

```
print pos2.
compute prob2=(pos2+1)/nperm.
print prob2/title=" factor 2 two tail probability".
end matrix.
```

Single-case AB design

The required files are *singlecaseAB.sps* (syntax for the macro) and *singlecase AB.sav* for the example data, which can also be seen in Table 4.10. To use the one-tailed test, the alternative hypothesis must be that the intervention increases the mean score. If the alternative is that the intervention decreases the mean score, then subtract all observations from a convenient round number larger than every observation. The original data for this example have been transformed in this way, all observations being subtracted from 50. The process was demonstrated for the single-case AB design in Chapter 4.

The phase designs all have an extra step at the beginning. In the datasheets we always code baseline or withdrawal as zero and intervention as 1, but we need to be able to use the phases as labels in the TOTALS and COUNTS matrices in the data matrix, so we increase the phase codes by 1 so they are 1 and 2 in the macro instead of 0 and 1. Then as usual we start the matrix language and collect the information from the datasheet. The DATA matrix has just two columns in this macro, one for the observations and the other for the phase.

```
set mxloop 5000.
compute phase = phase+1.
matrix.
get limits/variables=limits/missing=omit.
get data/variables=data phase/missing=omit.
```

First we calculate the test statistic for the actual experiment. It will be the difference between intervention and baseline means, so we need totals and counts for intervention and baseline. These can be calculated with exactly the same method as we used in the one-way design to get condition totals and counts. First we need to know how many rows of data, and we have to start the totals and counts at zero as usual. Then we step through the observations, adding each to the correct total and adding one to the correct count in the usual way.

```
compute nrows =limits(1).
compute totals={0;0}.
compute counts={0;0}.
loop row =1 to nrows.
```

```
compute totals(data(row,2))=totals(data(row,2))+data(row,1).
compute counts(data(row,2))=counts(data(row,2))+1.
end loop.
```

Now we calculate and print the test statistic for the actual experiment, using the same method as for the one-way design with two conditions.

```
compute means=totals/counts.
compute test=means(2)-means(1).
print test/title="test statistic".
```

Now we set the number of arrangements, set up a matrix to receive the results, and put the actual test statistic in the first place in the results matrix, all in exactly the same way as in previous macros.

```
compute nperm=2001.
compute results=uniform(nperm,1).
compute results(1,1)=test-test/1000000.
```

To perform the randomization for the phase designs, we have to choose a random number in the range determined by the minimum numbers of observations required for each phase. These minima follow the number of rows of data in the LIMITS matrix. First we choose a uniform random number (rand) between 0 and 1, then we have to use this to get a random number (inter) in the correct range for the intervention point. In our example data for this design, we have 35 rows of data, and we need a minimum of 5 for baseline and six for intervention. So the numbers temp1 and temp2 calculated below are 35–5–6+1 = 25 and 5+1 = 6. If we take just the whole number part of the random number temp1*rand using the trunc function, we get a random number between 0 and 24. Adding temp2 gives us a random number between 6 and 30, and this is the range of possible intervention points for this example. You may need to work through a few examples yourself to see that this method works for values of the minima required for baseline and intervention.

```
loop perm=2 to nperm.
compute rand=uniform(1,1).
compute temp1=limits(1)-limits(2)-limits(3)+1.
compute temp2=limits(2)+1.
compute inter=trunc(temp1*rand)+temp2.
```

Now we have the random intervention point for this arrangement, calculate the test statistic. This time we can't use the phase code to assign each observation to the correct total; we have to add up the observations before the intervention point, and then add those from the intervention onward.

```
compute totals={0;0}.
compute counts={0;0}.
loop row =1 to inter-1.              collect total and count for baseline
compute totals(1)=totals(1)+data(row,1).
compute counts(1)=counts(1)+1.
end loop.
loop row =inter to nrows.           and intervention
compute totals(2)=totals(2)+data(row,1).
compute counts(2)=counts(2)+1.
end loop.
compute means=totals/counts.        find the means and test statistic
compute test=means(2)-means(1).
compute results(perm,1)=test.       and put in the results matrix
end loop.                           next arrangement
```

Now we just have to compare the values from the reference set with our actual value. Because a one-tailed test is possible, we need the absolute values and two counts, just as in the one-way design with two conditions and the randomized blocks design with two conditions.

```
compute absres=abs(results).
compute pos1=0.
compute pos2=0.
loop k=2 to nperm.
do if results(k,1)>=results(1,1).
compute pos1=pos1+1.
end if.
do if absres(k,1)>=absres(1,1).
compute pos2=pos2+1.
end if.
end loop.
```

It only remains to print the counts and calculate and print one- and two-tailed probabilities, and this process is just the same as in other macros. After we end the matrix language, we restore the original phase codes.

```
print pos1/title="count of arrangement statistics at least *c*
as large".
compute prob1=(pos1+1)/nperm.
print prob1/title="one tail probability".
print pos2/title="count of arrangement statistics at least *c*
as large in abs value".
compute prob2=(pos2+1)/nperm.
```

```
print prob2/title="two tail probability".
end matrix.                          end of the matrix language
compute phase=phase-1.               restore the phase labels
execute.
```

Single-case ABA design

The required files are *singlecaseABA.sps* (syntax for the macro) and *singlecase ABA.sav* for the example data, which can also be seen in Table 4.12. To use the one-tailed test, the alternative hypothesis must be that the intervention increases the mean score. If the alternative is that the intervention decreases the mean score, then subtract all observations from a convenient round number larger than every observation.

This macro starts off just like the previous one. In fact, there are no differences until after we print the test statistic from the actual experiment.

```
set mxloop 5000.
compute phase = phase+1.
matrix.
get limits/variable=limits/missing=omit.
get data/variables=data phase/missing=omit.
compute nrows=limits(1).
compute totals={0;0}.
compute counts={0;0}.
loop row =1 to nrows.
compute totals(data(row,2))=totals(data(row,2))+data(row,1).
compute counts(data(row,2))=counts(data(row,2))+1.
end loop.
compute means=totals/counts.
compute test=means(2)-means(1).
print test/title="test statistic".
```

Now we need to find first how many possible intervention points there are, then how many intervention–withdrawal pairs. It is easy to check that the number of possible intervention points, NINTER, is as shown. However, to find the number of intervention–withdrawal pairs (NPAIRS) in terms of NINTER needs some knowledge of sequences and series. Checking a few special cases may convince you that it is correct below. We also need a matrix with NPAIRS rows and two columns to contain the possible intervention points (column 1) and withdrawal points (column 2). We call this matrix PAIRS and set it up by filling it with random numbers, a device we have used before. The contents will be overwritten with the intervention and withdrawal points as they are calculated.

```
compute ninter=limits(1)-limits(2)-limits(3)-limits(4)+1.
compute npairs=ninter*(ninter+1)/2.
compute pairs=uniform(npairs,2).
```

Now we step down the rows of the PAIRS matrix, calculating the intervention and withdrawal for each row. To do this again requires some knowledge of sequences and series, but trying out a few examples may convince you that it is correct below. Notice that we use the trunc function again. Remember that, for instance, trunc(4.3) is 4, but trunc(4.9) is also 4.

```
loop n=1 to npairs.
compute temp1=trunc(0.5+sqrt(2*n)).
compute temp2=n-0.5*temp1*(temp1-1).
compute pairs(n,1)=limits(1)-limits(3)-limits(4)+2-temp1.
compute pairs(n,2)=limits(1)-limits(4)+2-temp2.
end loop.
```

Now we start the rearrangements, 2000 as usual, plus one for the actual experiment. As usual, we set up a matrix with one column to receive the results and put the test statistic from the actual experiment at the top.

```
compute nperm=2001.
compute results=uniform(nperm,1).
compute results(1,1)=test-test/1000000.
```

For each rearrangement, we must choose a random number (RAND) that will identify the row to use from the PAIRS matrix. This random number must be in the range from 1 to the number of possible pairs we have, NPAIRS. From the chosen row, we read off the intervention point (column 1) and the withdrawal point (column 2).

```
loop perm=2 to nperm.
compute rand=trunc(npairs*uniform(1,1))+1.
compute interven=pairs(rand,1).
compute withdraw=pairs(rand,2).
```

To get the totals for the test statistic for this rearrangement, we can't use the phase codes, just as in the AB design; we have to step through the observations assigning to totals(1) before intervention and from withdrawal, and to totals(2) during intervention. Start the totals at zero, as usual.

```
compute totals={0;0}.
compute counts={0;0}.
loop row =1 to interven-1.
compute totals(1)=totals(1)+data(row,1).
compute counts(1)=counts(1)+1.
```

```
end loop.
loop row =interven to withdraw-1.
compute totals(2)=totals(2)+data(row,1).
compute counts(2)=counts(2)+1.
end loop.
loop row = withdraw to nrows.
compute totals(1)=totals(1)+data(row,1).
compute counts(1)=counts(1)+1.
end loop.
```

Once we have the totals and counts, the rest of the macro is the same as for the AB design.

```
compute means=totals/counts.
compute test=means(2)-means(1).
compute results(perm,1)=test.
end loop.
compute absres=abs(results).
compute pos1=0.
compute pos2=0.
loop k=2 to nperm.
do if results(k,1)>=results(1,1).
compute pos1=pos1+1.
end if.
do if absres(k,1)>=absres(1,1).
compute pos2=pos2+1.
end if.
end loop.
print pos1/title="count of arrangement statistics at least *c*
as large".
compute prob1=(pos1+1)/nperm.
print prob1/title="one tail probability".
print pos2/title="count of arrangement statistics at least *c*
as large in abs value".
compute prob2=(pos2+1)/nperm.
print prob2/title="two tail probability".
end matrix.
compute phase=phase-1.
execute.
```

Multiple baseline AB design

The required files are *multiplebaselineAB.sps* (syntax for the macro) and *multiplebaselineAB.sav* for the example data, which can also be seen in Table 4.13. To use the one-tailed test, the alternative hypotheses must be that the interventions increase the mean scores. If the alternatives are that the interventions decrease the mean scores, then subtract all observations from a convenient round number larger than every observation. This process is illustrated in the single-case AB example.

The macro begins in the same way as for the single-case AB design, but there is an extra column in the data matrix containing the codes for participants.

```
set mxloop 5000.
compute phase = phase+1.
matrix.
get limits/variable=limits/missing=omit.
get data/variables=data phase participant/missing=omit.
```

Collect the number of participants and the number of observations per participant. The number of rows of data can be calculated by multiplying them. We need to collect baseline and intervention totals and counts for each participant, so the TOTALS and COUNTS matrices must have two places for each participant.

```
compute nsubject=limits(1).
compute nrows =limits(2)*limits(1).
compute totals=make(nsubject,2,0).
compute counts=make(nsubject,2,0).
```

To get the baseline and intervention totals and counts, each observation has to be assigned to the correct total for its participant. Suppose we are on row 3 of the data, which is a baseline observation for participant 1. So data(row,3) will be 1 (for participant 1) and data(row,2) will be 1 (for baseline), so the observation in row 3 will increase total(1,1) by the number in data(3,1), which is the observation in row 3. In this way, all the totals and counts are accumulated.

```
loop row =1 to nrows.
compute totals(data(row,3),data(row,2))=*c*
totals(data(row,3),data(row,2))+data(row,1).
compute counts(data(row,3),data(row,2))=*c*
counts(data(row,3),data(row,2))+1.
end loop.
```

Once we have the totals, we have to get the test statistic. Getting the MEANS matrix is simple, exactly as before, but then we need to add up the differences between intervention and baseline means for all participants. Start TEST at zero, and work through the participants adding in each contribution.

```
compute means=totals/counts.
compute test=0.
loop k=1 to nsubject.
compute test=test+means(k,2)-means(k,1).
end loop.
print test/title="test statistic".
```

Setting the number of arrangements, setting up the results matrix, and putting the actual test statistic at the top are exactly as for the single-case design.

```
compute nperm=2001.
compute results=uniform(nperm,1).
compute results(1,1)=test-test/1000000.
```

Now we have to do the rearrangements. We calculate the number of possible intervention points (NINTER), which will be used to obtain a random number in the correct range. We start the test statistic at zero for each arrangement. It will receive a contribution from each participant. For each arrangement, we shall have to obtain the test statistic in the same way as we got it for the actual experiment. We can reuse the totals and counts matrices by multiplying by zero at the start of each arrangement. We collect up the contribution to the test statistic from each participant as we step through participants. However, we have to remember to start from the first observation for the current participant. If we are on participant k, previous participants occupy the first (k-1)*limit(2) rows of data, because there are limits(2) observations per participant.

```
loop perm=2 to nperm.
compute ninter=limits(2)−limits(3)−limits(4).
compute test=0.
```

Step through the participants. For each, we shall calculate intervention and baseline means, so for the current participant, start the totals, counts, and means at zero.

```
loop k= 1 to nsubject.
compute totals={0;0}.
compute counts={0;0}.
compute means={0;0}.
```

Find a random number between 1 and the number of possible intervention points, using the trunc function as before. From this, obtain the intervention point for the current participant. We first need to allow for the baseline observations, and there are limits(3) of those. Then we must remember that if we are on the second participant (for example), we have to allow for the observations from the first participant before deciding the row number for the intervention. This is why we add (k-1)*limits(2). If limits(2) is 15 as in our example, for participant 2, k–1=1 so the intervention row is 15+4+rand for our example. We also need to know the first and last rows of observations for the current participant (STARTROW and LASTROW).

```
compute rand=trunc(ninter*uniform(1,1))+1.
compute interven=rand+limits(3)+(k-1)*limits(2).
compute startrow=(k-1)*limits(2)+1.
compute lastrow=k*limits(2).
```

Now we can step down the rows of data for the current participant and obtain baseline and intervention totals, counts, and means. The difference between the means is added to the test statistic for the current participant. Then we move to the next participant. Then, when all participants are complete, put the test statistic in the next place in the RESULTS matrix and move to the next arrangement.

```
loop row =startrow to interven—1.
compute totals(1)=totals(1)+data(row,1).
compute counts(1)=counts(1)+1.
end loop.
loop row =interven to lastrow.
compute totals(2)=totals(2)+data(row,1).
compute counts(2)=counts(2)+1.
end loop.
compute means=totals/counts.
compute test=test+means(2)—means(1).
end loop.
compute results(perm,1)=test.
end loop.
```

Once we have the test statistics (reference set values) from all the arrangements, comparing with the one from the actual experiment and calculating and printing the probabilities are the same as for the single case.

```
compute absres=abs(results).
compute pos1=0.
compute pos2=0.
loop k=2 to nperm.
do if results(k,1)>=results(1,1).
compute pos1=pos1+1.
end if.
do if absres(k,1)>=absres(1,1).
compute pos2=pos2+1.
end if.
end loop.
print pos1/title="count of arrangement statistics at least *c*
as large".
compute prob1=(pos1+1)/nperm.
print prob1/title="one tail probability".
print pos2/title="count of arrangement statistics at least *c*
as large in abs value".
compute prob2=(pos2+1)/nperm.
```

```
print prob2/title="two tail probability".
end matrix.
compute phase=phase-1.
execute.
```

Multiple baseline ABA design

The required files are *multiplebaselineABA.sps* (syntax for the macro) and *multiplebaselineABA.sav* for the example data, which can also be seen in Table 4.14. To use the one-tailed test, the alternative hypotheses must be that the interventions increase the mean scores. If the alternatives are that the interventions decrease the mean scores, then subtract all observations from a convenient round number larger than every observation. This process is illustrated in the single-case AB example.

This macro begins in exactly the same way as the multiple baseline AB macro.

```
set mxloop 5000.
compute phase = phase+1.
matrix.
get limits/variable=limits/missing=omit.
get data/variables=data phase participant/missing=omit.
compute nsubject=limits(1).
compute nrows =limits(2)*limits(1).
compute totals=make(nsubject,2,0).
compute counts=make(nsubject,2,0).
loop row =1 to nrows.
compute totals(data(row,3),data(row,2))=*c*
totals(data(row,3),data(row,2))+data(row,1).
compute counts(data(row,3),data(row,2))=*c*
counts(data(row,3),data(row,2))+1.
end loop.
compute means=totals/counts.
compute test=0.
loop k=1 to nsubject.
compute test=test+means(k,2)-means(k,1).
end loop.
print test/title= "test statistic".
compute nperm=2001.
compute results=uniform(nperm,1).
compute results(1,1)=test-test/1000000.
```

Just as in the single-case ABA design, we need to find first how many possible intervention points there are, then how many intervention–withdrawal pairs. It is easy to check that the number of possible intervention points, NINTER, is as shown. We use the same method of finding the number of intervention–withdrawal pairs as we did for the single-case ABA design. Also, we need a matrix with NPAIRS rows and two columns to contain the possible intervention points (column 1) and withdrawal points (column 2), just as in the single-case ABA design. We call this matrix PAIRS and set it up by filling it with random numbers, a device we have used before. The contents will be overwritten with the intervention and withdrawal points as they are calculated.

```
compute ninter=limits(2)-limits(3)-limits(4)-limits(5)+1.
compute npairs=ninter*(ninter+1)/2.
compute pairs=uniform(npairs,2).
loop n=1 to npairs.
compute temp1=trunc(0.5+sqrt(2*n)).
compute temp2=n-0.5*temp1*(temp1-1).
compute pairs(n,1)=limits(2)-limits(4)-limits(5)+2-temp1.
compute pairs(n,2)=limits(2)-limits(5)+2-temp2.
end loop.
```

As in the single-case ABA design, set the number of arrangements, and make a matrix to receive the results and put the actual value from the experiment at the top.

```
compute nperm=2001.
compute results=uniform(nperm,1).
compute results(1,1)=test-test/1000000.
```

Now we start the rearrangements. For each new arrangement, we need to start the test statistic off at zero. As we step through the participants, a contribution will be added from each of them.

```
loop perm=2 to nperm.
compute test=0.
```

In each arrangement, we step through the participants. For each participant, we must choose a random number and use it to identify the intervention–withdrawal pair just as in the single-case ABA design. Then, because we have several participants, we need to find the row of the DATA matrix where the current participant's observations start (STARTROW) and finish (LASTROW). This is a multiple of the number of observations per participant.

```
loop k= 1 to nsubject.
compute rand=trunc(npairs*uniform(1,1))+1.
compute interven=pairs(rand,1)+(k-1)*limits(2).
compute withdraw=pairs(rand,2)+(k-1)*limits(2).
compute startrow=(k-1)*limits(2)+1.
compute lastrow=k*limits(2).
```

Now we are ready to find the intervention and baseline–withdrawal means for the current participant. This is just like the single-case ABA design, except that we start at the first row for this participant rather than row 1, and end at the last row for this participant.

```
compute totals={0;0}.
compute counts={0;0}.
compute means={0;0}.
loop row =startrow to interven-1.
compute totals(1)=totals(1)+data(row,1).
compute counts(1)=counts(1)+1.
end loop.
loop row =interven to withdraw-1.
compute totals(2)=totals(2)+data(row,1).
compute counts(2)=counts(2)+1.
end loop.
loop row =withdraw to lastrow.
compute totals(1)=totals(1)+data(row,1).
compute counts(1)=counts(1)+1.
end loop.
```

Find the intervention and baseline–withdrawal means for the current participant, and add the difference to the test statistic for this arrangement. Then move to the next participant.

```
compute means=totals/counts.
compute test=test+means(2)-means(1).
end loop.
```

Once we have the test statistic for this arrangement (the total of the participants' contributions for this arrangement), save it and move to the next arrangement.

```
compute results(perm,1)=test.
end loop.
```

From now on, it's just the same as for the other phase designs.

```
compute absres=abs(results).
compute pos1=0.
compute pos2=0.
loop k=2 to nperm.
do if results(k,1)>=results(1,1).
compute pos1=pos1+1.
end if.
do if absres(k,1)>=absres(1,1).
compute pos2=pos2+1.
end if.
end loop.
print pos1/title="count of arrangement statistics at least *c*
as large".
```

```
compute prob1=(pos1+1)/nperm.
print prob1/title="one tail probability".
print pos2/title="count of arrangement statistics at least *c*
as large in abs value".
compute prob2=(pos2+1)/nperm.
print prob2/title="two tail probability".
end matrix.
compute phase=phase-1.
execute.
```

A design to test ordinal predictions

The macro is *ordereffects.sps*, and the example data file is *ordereffects.sav*, which can also be seen in Table 4.15. The coding should make the predicted correlation positive. The example data can be replaced by any other suitable example, but the variable names should be retained.

The macro starts in the same way as all the others, and there are two columns in the DATA matrix, which are the observations and the predicted order. As in most other macros, we call the number of rows of data nrows.

```
set mxloop=5000.
matrix.
get limits/variables=limits/missing=omit.
get data/variables=data predict/missing=omit
compute nrows=limits(1).
```

The test statistic is the sum of products of the observations with their predicted order, and we collect this from the actual data first, as in all the macros. Start the sum of products at zero, and step down the rows of data, adding in the contribution from each. Print the result.

```
compute sumprod=0.
loop row=1 to nrows.
compute sumprod=sumprod+data(row,1)*data(row,2).
end loop.
print sumprod/title="sum of products".
```

Set the number of arrangements, make a matrix to receive the reference set values, and put the value from the actual experiment at the top, all just as in previous macros.

```
compute nperm=2001.
compute results=uniform(nperm,1).
compute results(1,1)=sumprod-sumprod/1000000.
```

We can rearrange the observations, or we can rearrange the predicted order; it makes no difference, but we have chosen to rearrange the observations. The method is just the same as used for the one-way design.

```
loop perm=2 to nperm.
loop row=1 to nrow.
compute k=trunc(uniform(1,1)*(ncase-row+1))+row.
compute temp=data(row,1).
compute data(row,1)=data(k,1).
compute data(k,1)=temp.
end loop.
```

For each arrangement, start the sum of products at zero, and step through the rearranged data to get the test statistic for this arrangement. Put it in the next place in the RESULTS matrix.

```
compute sumprod=0.
loop row=1 to nrows.
compute sumprod=sumprod+data(row,1)*data(row,2).
end loop.
compute results(perm,1)=sumprod.
end loop.                        move to the next arrangement
```

The comparison of the actual test statistic to the other 2000 values in the reference set, calculating and printing the probability, is just as for other macros.

```
compute pos=0.
loop k=2 to nperm.
do if results(k,1)>=results(1,1).
compute pos=pos+1.
end if.
end loop.
print pos/title="count of arrangement sums of products *c*
at least as large".
compute prob=(pos+1)/nperm.
print prob/title="probability".
end matrix.
```

Appendix 3: Excel macros

Introduction

The first section, "Running a Macro in Excel," should be useful to anyone wanting to use our macros to analyze their data. The remainder of this appendix, starting with the section "Editing a Macro in Excel," is needed only if you want to understand the macros to modify them or write your own. If you just want to use our macros as they are, you should skip these later sections.

Running a macro in Excel

Excel keeps data and macros all in the workbook. All our examples are saved as macro-enabled workbooks with the extension .xlsm, for example oneway.xlsm. When you open these workbooks, you may still have to click **Enable macros** using **Macro Security** in the **Code** group of the **Developer** tab on the menu bar. You need to have suitable data (such as our example data) in the active datasheet. When you open the workbooks, they do already have the data from an appropriate example in the active datasheet. To run a macro, select the **Developer** tab from the menu bar, and click the **Macros** button. A dialog box like Figure A3.1 *Excel Dialog Box A3.1* appears. If there is only one macro stored in the workbook, just click **Run**. All our workbooks contain just one macro, but in general if there is more than one, select the one you want and click **Run**. In a few minutes, the results appear in the datasheet as shown in Figure A3.2 *Excel Output A3.1*, but remember that as we take a random sample from the reference set, your results in column L will not be identical to ours.

To run our macros, take them from the book Web site (http://www. researchmethodsarena.com/9780415886932). After trying out the macros with the example data, edit the data to replace the example data with your own, but retain the names for the variables. In some cases (the oneway design is one), you also need to edit the name ranges as shown in the

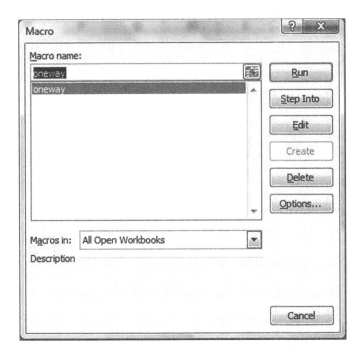

Figure A3.1 *Excel Dialog Box A3.1.* Running a macro.

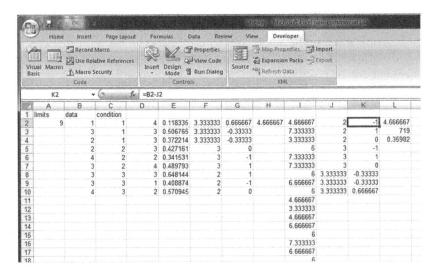

Figure A3.2 *Excel Output A3.1.* The one-way single-case example.

next section of this chapter. Where this is needed, instructions are provided in Chapter 5.

Editing name ranges in a macro in Excel

If names are used by an Excel macro, the ranges must be correct for the
data. Ranges can easily be edited when new data are to be used; just follow these steps.

1. On the **Formulas** tab, select **Name Manager** in the **Defined Names**
   group. The Name Manager window opens as shown in Figure A3.3
   Excel Dialog Box A3.2 (this is the window for the *multiplebaselineAB*
   design example).
2. Several names on the list will have a range ending in the last row of
   data. For the example shown, the names DATA and LEVEL have ranges
   ending in 31, the last data row for this example. These are the ones to
   edit.
3. Select the first of them (DATA in the window shown), and click **Edit**.

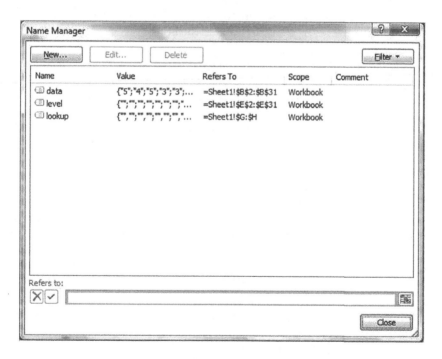

Figure A3.3 *Excel Dialog Box A3.2.* The Name Manager window for the
multiplebaselineAB example.

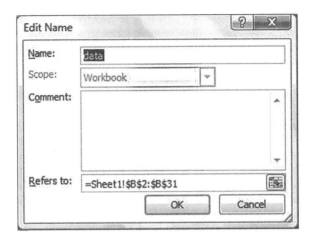

Figure A3.4 Excel Dialog Box A3.3. The Edit Name window for the multiplebaselineAB example.

4. This opens the Edit Name window shown in Figure A3.4 *Excel Dialog Box A3.3*. Click in the **Refers to** box at the bottom, and change 31 (the bottom row of the example data) to the bottom row of your new data. Click **OK**.
5. Back in the **Name Manager** dialog box, select the next name (LEVEL) and **Edit** in the same way. There are no more ranges to edit for this example. Figure A3.5 *Excel Dialog Box A3.4* shows the Name Manager window when we had finished editing names for a new set of data that finished on row 26. Click the **Close** button at the bottom.

You can now run the macro with the new data.

Editing a macro in Excel

The remainder of this appendix need be read only by those wishing to adapt our macros or write their own. If you are writing your own, you should also consult Chapter 8. Excel macros are written in Visual Basic. You can edit one by clicking the **Edit** button in Excel Dialog Box A3.1. The Visual Basic code is then displayed in a new window (see Figure A3.6 *Excel Visual Basic window A3.1*). If you want to try out some ideas without destroying your original macro, select all the macro code and copy to the clipboard using Ctrl C. Now enter a new macro name (something like "testing" might be appropriate), and click the **Create** button. Paste the code in between the Sub and End Sub lines. Now you have a copy you can try things out in, while the original remains intact with its original name.

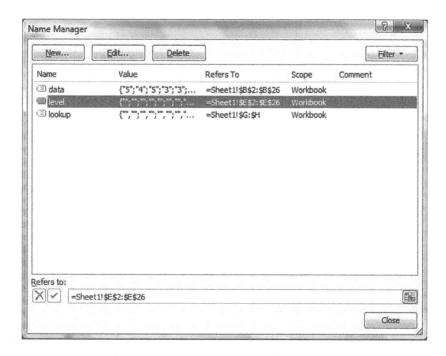

Figure A3.5 *Excel Dialog Box A3.4.* The Name Manager window with range editing complete.

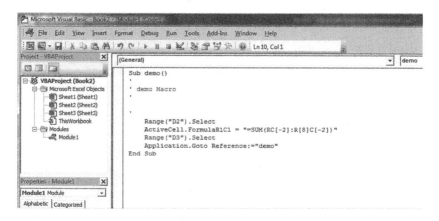

Figure A3.6 *Excel Visual Basic window A3.1.*

Writing a macro in Excel

To write a macro in an Excel workbook, click the **Developer** tab and then the **Macro** button in the **Code** group. A dialog box opens, and if you type a name (for example, "demo") in the **Macro name** box, the **Create** button becomes available. If you click **Create**, the Visual Basic edit window opens with the cursor blinking between the first and last lines of the macro. The first line is Sub demo() for our example where we used the name demo, and the last line is End Sub. You can write and edit your code in this window and run it by clicking Run on the menu bar.

If there are already macros in the workbook, when you open the macro dialog box, the first will be in the **Macro name** box (Figure A3.1 *Excel Dialog Box A3.1*). To start a new macro, just type the name for your new one in the **Macro name** box instead of the one that is already there.

Excel offers a shortcut to writing macros using the **Record Macro** button on the **Developer** tab. When you click the **Record Macro** button, you will see a dialog box where you need to type a name for your macro (we typed "demo" for this example). Click **OK**, and thereafter all operations you perform will be recorded in Visual Basic until you click the **Stop recording** button. In the Visual Basic window, you can now see the commands that effected the operations you performed. All we did for this example was type =Sum(B2:B10) in cell D2. Then we clicked **Stop recording**. In Figure A3.6 *Excel Visual Basic window A3.1*, you can see the result. This example shows that Visual Basic is not a concise language, and also that using the **Record Macro** button may save a lot of effort.

Understanding the macros

Introduction and general notes

In this section, we list the syntax for the Excel macros with added notes. We begin with a few general notes that apply to nearly every macro, and then proceed to the annotated listings.

All the macros follow this pattern.

1. Begin by clearing the datasheet columns to be used. Then set up some integer variables for the number of observations (also participants, conditions, or blocks where needed), and for counting arrangements. We also need an integer to denote the last row of data.
2. Make a copy of the data so that they can be rearranged without disturbing the original. This step is not part of the phase design macros. Instead, for phase designs, it is necessary to make a lookup table and a column of identification numbers for the observations.

3. The main part of the macro performs the rearrangements and calculates the rearrangement test statistics to form the reference set.
4. Find the test statistic for the actual experiment.
5. Compare values in the reference set with the actual test statistic.
6. Finally two-tailed (and one-tailed, where appropriate) test probabilities are calculated.

Except for phase designs, rearrangements are performed by using a column of random numbers that is then sorted into order, carrying the data copy along into the new order. In the phase designs, we use a lookup table to choose intervention points at random from those available.

The Excel Autofill function, which enables us to copy a formula down a column, appears in Visual Basic as Autofill. Here is an example:

```
Selection.AutoFill Destination:=Range("F2:F" & lastrow$),_
Type:=xlFillDefault.
```

This will copy the selected cell from F2 down column F to the last row of data.

The underscore, _, can be used as a continuation symbol for long commands, but it can't be used just anywhere. The command needs to be broken after a comma, an ampersand (&), an equals sign (=), or some other suitable break point, then the underscore will continue it onto the next line. As we remarked, Visual Basic is not concise, and the width of the page doesn't always enable us to get to a suitable break before overrunning, so we use *c* as our continuation symbol. When you see *c* in what follows, it is not part of the code but just shows that we have overrun but not in a place where we can use the underscore to continue.

Visual Basic uses R and C to denote the row and column currently being worked on. This is called the active cell. Previous rows and columns are denoted like R[-2], which denotes the second row above the current one. C[-3] denotes the third column before the current one. So if we are currently working with column K, C[-3] refers to column H.

To obtain the test statistics, we often use the functions SUMIF and COUNTIF. Here is an example:

```
Sumif(condition,RC[-3],arrange).
```

The first argument, condition, will be checked against the second argument, RC[-3]. The third argument, arrange, names the variable that will be summed. So, in this example, a sum for each "condition" of the variable "arrange" will be formed. Further details of these functions can be found in the Excel Help file.

To store the test statistics from the rearrangements in a column, we use Insert Shift, which inserts the active cell at the top of the selected column, pushing values already in the column down one cell. Here is what it looks like:

```
Selection.Insert Shift:=xlDown
Selection.PasteSpecial Paste:=xlValues.
```

We include the step numbers (but not the headings) from the beginning of this section. There is some commentary between blocks of code as well as extra comments in bold next to some lines of code. At the start of each macro, we briefly list the columns used and their contents.

One-way design (single-case or small-n)

The required file is *oneway.xlsm*, which also contains the data for the single-case example. You can look at the example data in Tables 4.1 and 4.2. The data in the workbook may be replaced with any other example, but the name ranges must be edited as explained in the "Editing Name Ranges in a Macro in Excel" section of this chapter. Leave the variable names unchanged. Here is the column list.

A–C: Original data entered by user
D: Copy of B for rearrangement
E: Random numbers
F: Rearrangement condition means
G: Rearrangement residuals
H: Current RSS
I: Saved RSS from rearrangements
J: Actual condition means
K: Actual RSS
L: Final results

1. Clear the columns to be used. Note that columns A to C are used for the experimental data and column D will be used to contain rearranged data. If you check the Names Manager for this workbook, you find that column D has a name, "arrange," so that the macro can refer to the rearranged data.

We also need some integers to denote the number of observations and the last row of data and for counting arrangements. Because the first row of the datasheet carries the column names, the last row of data is not the same as the number of observations. The number of observations is read from cell A2 in the datasheet.

```
Sub oneway()
Columns("E:O").ClearContents        clear area to be used
Dim j As Integer                    for counting arrangements
Dim last_i As Integer               number of observations
last_i = Range("A2")
Dim lastrow$                        row number for bottom of columns of
                                    data and arrangements

lastrow$ = last_i + 1
```

2. Now copy the observations from column B into column D, where they will be rearranged.

```
Range("B2:B" & lastrow$).Select
Selection.Copy                      copy the observations so they can
                                    be rearranged
Range("D2").Select
ActiveSheet.Paste
```

3. Now we do the rearrangements and calculate the test statistic for each one. The first command sets the number of rearrangements at 2000 (you can easily change this, but if you do, be sure to change the divisors for the probability near the end).

In column E, we put a column of random numbers (which will be uniformly spread over the interval 0 to 1). Then, when we select columns D and E and sort them on column E, we shall have the observations arranged in random order.

```
For j = 1 To 2000                   loop for 2000
                                    rearrangements
Range("E2").Select                  select E2
ActiveCell.FormulaR1C1 = "=Rand()"  and put in a random
                                    number
Selection.AutoFill _                and fill down the rest of
Destination:= Range("E2:E" & _ lastrow$),    column E
Type:= xlFillDefault
Range("D2:E" & lastrow$).Select     select columns D and E
Selection.Sort Key1:=Range("E2"),_  sort on column E so we
Order1:=xlAscending, Header:= xlGuess,_   have a rearrangement
OrderCustom:=1, MatchCase:=False,_  of column D
Orientation:= xlTopToBottom
```

Now that we have a rearrangement, we need to find the test statistic. As a first step, we fill column F with the condition means. The condition codes are in column C (the third column before F), and we find the mean for each condition using the rearranged data in column D. Do the calculation for F2, and fill down the rest of column F. Sumif gets the condition totals, and Countif gets the number of observations in each condition.

```
Range("F2").Select
ActiveCell.FormulaR1C1 = "=Sumif(condition,*c*
RC[-3],arrange)/Countif(condition,RC[-3])"
Selection.AutoFill Destination:=Range("F2:F" & _
lastrow$), Type:=xlFillDefault
```

To find the RSS, we find the residual for each rearranged observation, then sum the squared residuals. The residual is the rearranged observation minus its condition mean. Calculate the first residual in G2, then fill down column G. Calculate the RSS in H2.

```
Range("G2").Select
ActiveCell.FormulaR1C1 = "=RC[-3]-RC[-1]"
Selection.AutoFill Destination:=Range("G2:G" & lastrow$),_
Type:=xlFillDefault
Range("H2").Select
ActiveCell.FormulaR1C1 = "=Sumsq(C[-1])"
```

Then the RSS for this arrangement must be stored. It will be copied into the top of column I, all previous values being moved down one row. Then we move on to the next arrangement.

```
Selection.Copy
Range("I2").Select
Selection.Insert Shift:=xlDown
Selection.PasteSpecial Paste:=xlValues
Next                                        next arrangement
```

4. Now we find the test statistic for the actual data in exactly the same way as for the rearrangements. The condition means for the actual data are put in column J (calculate J2 and fill down).

```
Range("J2").Select
ActiveCell.FormulaR1C1 = "=Sumif(condition,*c*
RC[-7],data)/Countif(condition,RC[-7])"
Selection.AutoFill Destination:=Range("J2:J" & lastrow$),_
Type:=xlFillDefault
Range("K2").Select
ActiveCell.FormulaR1C1 = "=RC[-9]-*c*
RC[-1]"                            fill in the actual residuals
Selection.AutoFill Destination:=Range("K2:K" & lastrow$),_
```

```
Type:=xlFillDefault
Range("L2").FormulaR1C1 = *c*
"=Sumsq(C[-1])"                              actual RSS goes into L2
```

5 and 6. Now we must count the cases where the rearrangement RSS is at least as small as the actual RSS. The count goes in L3. The probability of a result at least as extreme as the actual experiment is the count in L3 divided by 2001. Remember to change this divisor if you change the number of arrangements.

```
Range("L3").FormulaR1C1 = "=Countif(C[-3]:C[-3], *c*
""<=""&R[-1]C)"
                        count the cases where the arrangement
                        RSS is <= actual
Range("L4").FormulaR1C1 = "=(R[-1]C+1)/(2000+1)"
                        probability of a result at least as
                        extreme as the actual one
End Sub
```

One-way design (single-case or small-n) with just two conditions

The required file is *onewaytwoconditions.xlsm*, which also contains the data for the small-*n* example (which can be seen in Table 4.3). The data may be deleted and replaced with any other suitable data, but leave the variable names unchanged. Here is the column list.

A–C: Original data entered by user
D: Copy of B
E: Random numbers
F: Rearrangement and actual condition means and test statistics
G: Stored arrangement test statistics
H: Stored absolute values of test statistics SS
I: Final results

1 and 2. This macro begins in exactly the same way as the previous one, clearing the area to be used, setting up integers, reading the number of observations from A2, and copying the observations into column D for rearranging.

```
Sub onewaytwoconditions()
Columns("E:O").ClearContents
Dim j As Integer
Dim last_i As Integer
```

```
last_i = Range("A2")
Dim lastrow$
lastrow$ = last_i + 1
Range("B2:B" & lastrow$).Select
Selection.Copy
Range("D2").Select
ActiveSheet.Paste
```

3. Then we start the rearrangements and put random numbers in column E as before, then sort the random numbers, carrying along the observations so we have a rearrangement, all just as in the previous macro.

```
For j = 1 To 2000
Range("E2").Select
ActiveCell.FormulaR1C1 = "=Rand()"
Selection.AutoFill Destination:=Range("E2:E" & lastrow$), _
Type:=xlFillDefault
Range("D2:E" & lastrow$).Select
Selection.Sort Key1:=Range("E2"), Order1:=xlAscending, _
Header:=xlGuess, OrderCustom:=1, MatchCase:=False, _
Orientation:=xlTopToBottom
```

This time, the test statistic is the difference between condition means. We put the condition 2 mean in F2 and the condition 1 mean in F3, then F2–F3 into F4. This is the test statistic for this arrangement.

```
Range("F2").Select
ActiveCell.FormulaR1C1 = "=Sumif(C[-3]:C[-3], ""=2"", *c*
[-2]:C[-2])/Countif(C[-3]:C[-3],""=2"")"
Range("F3").Select
ActiveCell.FormulaR1C1 = "=Sumif(C[-3]:C[-3], ""=1"", *c*
C[-2]:C[-2])/Countif(C[-3]:C[-3],""=1"")"
Range("F4").Select
ActiveCell.FormulaR1C1 = "=R[-2]C-R[-1]C"
```

Then we have to store the test statistic, so we copy it into the top of column G and move all previous values down one row, just as we did with column I in the previous macro.

```
Selection.Copy
Range("G2").Select
Selection.Insert Shift:=xlDown
Selection.PasteSpecial Paste:=xlValues
```

Because this macro allows both one- and two-tailed tests, we now put the absolute value of the test statistic into F5 and copy it to the top of column H, moving all previous values down one row. Then move on to the next arrangement.

```
Range("F5").Select
ActiveCell.FormulaR1C1 = "=ABS(R[-1]C)"
Selection.Copy
Range("H2").Select
Selection.Insert Shift:=xlDown
Selection.PasteSpecial Paste:=xlValues
Next
```

4. Now find the test statistic and its absolute value for the actual data. The condition 2 mean for the actual data goes into F6, and the condition 1 mean into F7. The test statistic goes into F8, and its absolute value into F9.

```
Range("F6").Select
ActiveCell.FormulaR1C1 = "=Sumif(C[-3]:C[-3], ""=2"", *C*
C[-4]:C[-4])/Countif(C[-3]:C[-3],""=2"")"
Range("F7").Select
ActiveCell.FormulaR1C1 = "=Sumif(C[-3]:C[-3], ""=1"", *C*
C[-4]:C[-4])/Countif(C[-3]:C[-3],""=1"")"
Range("F8").Select
ActiveCell.FormulaR1C1 = "=R[-2]C-R[-1]C"
Range("F9").Select
ActiveCell.FormulaR1C1 = "=ABS(R[-1]C)"
```

5 and 6. Now we collect up the results in column I. The test statistic goes into I2. The count of arrangement values at least as large goes into I3, and the one-tailed probability into I4. Then into I5 goes the absolute value of the test statistic, followed by the count of absolute values at least as large in I6 and the two-tailed probability in I7.

```
Range("I2").FormulaR1C1 = "=R[6]C[-3]"
Range("I3").FormulaR1C1 = _
"=Countif(C[-2]:C[-2],"">=""&R[5]C[-3])"
Range("I4").FormulaR1C1 = "=(R[-1]C+1)/(2000+1)"
Range("I5").FormulaR1C1 = "=R[4]C[-3]"
Range("I6").FormulaR1C1 = _
"=Countif(C[-1]:C[-1],"">=""&R[3]C[-3])"
Range("I7").FormulaR1C1 = "=(R[-1]C+1)/(2000+1)"
End Sub
```

A randomized blocks design (single-case or small-n repeated measures)

The required file is *randomizedblocks.xlsm*, which also contains the data for the single-case example (which can be seen in Table 4.4). The example data may be deleted and replaced with any other suitable data, but in this case the name ranges must be edited as explained in the "One-Way Design (Single-Case or Small-*n*) With Just Two Conditions" section of this chapter. If you check the Names Manager for this workbook, you find that column F has a name, "arrange," so that the macro can refer to the rearranged data. Leave the variable names unchanged. Here is a column list.

A–D: Original data entered by user
E: Grand mean of observations
F: Copy of B
G: Random numbers
H: Rearrangement condition means
I: Rearrangement block means
J: Rearrangement residuals
K: Current RSS
L: Saved RSS from rearrangements
M: Actual condition means
N: Actual block means
O: Actual residuals
P: Final results

1. We begin in the same way as the previous macros, by clearing the columns to be used, setting up integers, reading the number of observations from A2, and calculating the last row of data.

```
Sub randomizedblocks()
Columns("E:P").ClearContents
Dim j As Integer
Dim lastobs$
lastobs = Range("A2")
Dim lastrow$
lastrow$ = lastobs + 1
```

Because the mean of all the observations (called the grand mean) will be used to calculate the residuals for both the actual and rearranged observations, we begin by calculating the grand mean in E2 and copy it down to the last row of data.

```
Range("E2").Select
ActiveCell.FormulaR1C1 = "=SUM(C[-3])/Count(C[-3])"
Selection.AutoFill Destination:=Range("E2:E" & lastrow$)
```

2. Now we make a copy of the observations that will then be rearranged. The copy will go in column F because column C contains condition codes, column D contains block codes, and column E contains the grand mean.

```
Range("B2:B" & lastrow$).Select
Selection.Copy
Range("F2").Select
ActiveSheet.Paste
```

3. Now we set the number of rearrangements, perform the rearrange-ments, and obtain and store the test statistic for each one. For this design we need to rearrange observations within each block. This can be achieved by adding the block number from column D to the random number cor-responding to each (copied) observation. So the block 1 observations will have random numbers smaller than the block 2 observations, which will have random numbers smaller than the block 3 observations, and so on. We then select columns F and G, containing the copied observations and random numbers plus block numbers, and sort on column G.

```
For j = 1 To 2000
Range("G2").Select
ActiveCell.FormulaR1C1 = "=RAND()+RC[-3]"
Selection.AutoFill Destination:=Range("G2:G" & lastrow$), _
Type:=xlFillDefault
Range("F2:G" & lastrow$).Select
Selection.Sort Key1:=Range("G2"), Order1:=xlAscending, _
Header:=xlGuess, OrderCustom:=1, MatchCase:=False,_
Orientation:=xlTopToBottom
```

Now that we have a rearrangement, we need to find the test statistic. This time the residual is the observation minus the condition mean, minus the block mean, plus the grand mean. In column H we put the condition means, obtained using Sumif and Countif as in the oneway design.

```
Range("H2").Select
ActiveCell.FormulaR1C1 = "=SUMIF(condition,*c*
RC[-5],arrange)/COUNTIF(condition,RC[-5])"
Selection.AutoFill Destination:=Range("H2:H" & *c*
lastrow$)
```

Then in column I put the block means, obtained in a similar way.

```
Range("I2").Select
ActiveCell.FormulaR1C1 = "=SUMIF(block,*c*
RC[-5],arrange)/COUNTIF(block,RC[-5])"
Selection.AutoFill Destination:=Range("I2:I" & *c*
lastrow$)
```

The grand mean is in column E, with a copy in each row. Now we calcu-late the residual for each rearranged observation (do the first one in J2 and fill down).

```
Range("J2").Select
ActiveCell.FormulaR1C1 = "=RC[-4]-RC[-2]-*c*
RC[-1]+RC[-5]"
Selection.AutoFill Destination:=Range("J2:J" & *c*
lastrow$)
```

To find the RSS for this arrangement, we square and add the residuals, then store at the top of column L, pushing previous values down one row. Then we can go to the next arrangement.

```
Range("K2").Select
ActiveCell.FormulaR1C1 = "=SUMSQ(C[-1])"
Selection.Copy
Range("L2").Select
Selection.Insert Shift:=xlDown
Selection.PasteSpecial Paste:=xlValues
Next
```

4. Once we have all the arrangement statistics, we need to find the RSS for the actual experiment. We do this in the same way, putting condition means in column M and block means in column N, and using the grand mean from column E. The residuals go into column O.

```
Range("M2").Select
ActiveCell.FormulaR1C1 = "=SUMIF(condition,*c*
RC[-10],data)/COUNTIF(condition,RC[-10])"
Selection.AutoFill Destination:=Range("M2:M" & lastrow$)
Range("N2").Select
ActiveCell.FormulaR1C1 = "=SUMIF(block,*c*
RC[-10],data)/COUNTIF(block,RC[-10])"
Selection.AutoFill Destination:=Range("N2:N" & lastrow$)
Range("O2").Select
ActiveCell.FormulaR1C1 = "=RC[-13]-RC[-2]-RC[-1]+RC[-10]"
Selection.AutoFill Destination:=Range("O2:O" & lastrow$)
```

Now find the sum of squared residuals (the RSS) for the actual data and put it in P2.

```
Range("P2").Select
ActiveCell.FormulaR1C1 = "=SUMSQ(C[-1])"
```

5 and 6. Now in P3, put the count of arrangements statistics at least as small as the actual one in P2. Divide by 2001 to get the probability in P4.

```
Range("P3").Select
ActiveCell.FormulaR1C1 = _
"=COUNTIF(C[-4]:C[-4],""<=""&R[-1]C)"
Range("P4").Select
ActiveCell.FormulaR1C1 = "=(R[-1]C+1)/(2000+1)"
End Sub
```

A randomized blocks design with two conditions (single-case or small-n repeated measures)

The workbook *randomizedblockstwoconditions.xlsm* contains the macro and the single-case example data (which can be seen in Table 4.6). To use with other data, just delete the data in cells A2 to D15 and enter the new data. Keep the variable names the same, and remember that if you are using a one-tailed test, the condition with higher predicted mean must be coded 2. This macro demonstrates a different approach from the previous ones and does not use step 2, copying the data for rearrangement. Here is the column list.

A–D: Original data entered by user
E: Random numbers
F: 1s and 0s corresponding to a rearrangement
G: Column F multiplied by column B
H: Rearrangement difference between condition totals (the test statistic)
I: Saved test statistics from rearrangements
J: Absolute values of I
K: Column B multiplied by (column C–1)
L: Actual difference between condition totals and its absolute value
M: Final results

1. As usual we begin by clearing the columns to be used and setting up integers. The number of blocks is in A2 and from this we can calculate the number of rows of data, since each of the 2 conditions occurs once in each block.

```
Sub randomizedblockstwoconditions()
Columns("E:M").ClearContents
Dim j As Integer
Dim lastblock As Integer
lastblock = Range("A2")
Dim lastrow$
lastrow$ = 2 * lastblock + 1
```

3. Now we set the number of rearrangements and put random numbers in column E.

```
For j = 1 To 2000
Range("E2").Select
ActiveCell.FormulaR1C1 = "=RAND()"
Selection.AutoFill Destination:=Range("E2:E" & lastrow$)
```

For this design, we need to rearrange the observations or conditions within blocks. Because there are only two observations in each block, all we have to do is decide which comes first in the rearrangement. It's easiest to rearrange conditions. The test statistic will be the difference between condition means (because we have only two conditions). This time we show you a method that does not need us to use names, so that replacing the example data with your own data does not involve editing name ranges. This is how we do it. In F2, put a 1 if the random number in E2 is > 0.5; otherwise, put a zero. Then, in F3, put a 0 if F2 has a 1, and a 1 if F2 has a 0. Then copy F2:F3 down the column to the last row of data.

```
Range("F2").Select
ActiveCell.FormulaR1C1 = "=IF(RC[-1]>0.5,0,1)"
Range("F3").Select
ActiveCell.FormulaR1C1 = "=1-R[-1]C"
Range("F2:F3").Select
Selection.AutoFill Destination:=Range("F2:F" & lastrow$)
```

Now in F we have a column of 1s and 0s corresponding to a rearrangement of the conditions. If we multiply column F by the data in column B and add the result, we shall have the sum of those observations that were assigned a 1 in the rearrangement. If we double this sum and subtract the total of observations, we shall have the difference between condition totals for the rearrangement. Comparing the difference between condition totals for the actual and rearranged data is equivalent to comparing the difference between means, and we use totals. The product of columns F and B goes into column G, and the difference between condition totals goes into H2.

```
Range("G2").Select
ActiveCell.FormulaR1C1 = "=RC[-5]*RC[-1]"
Selection.AutoFill Destination:=Range("G2:G" & lastrow$)
Range("H2").Select
ActiveCell.FormulaR1C1 = "=2*SUM(C[-1]:C[-1])*c*
-SUM(C[-6]:C[-6])"
```

Store the test statistic at the top of column I, pushing values from previous arrangements down one row. Then go to the next arrangement.

```
Selection.Copy
Range("I2").Select
Selection.Insert Shift:=xlDown
Selection.PasteSpecial Paste:=xlValues
Next
```

Because we have only two conditions and a directional alternative hypothesis is possible, we need to obtain the absolute values of the arrangement test statistics. These will go into column J, and we fill down to the last row of arrangement statistics.

```
lastperm$ = j
Range("J2").Select
ActiveCell.FormulaR1C1 = "=ABS(RC[-1])"
Selection.AutoFill Destination:=Range("J2:J" & lastperm$)
```

4. Now we have to find the test statistic and its absolute value for the actual experiment. We subtract 1 from the condition codes in column C so that we multiply the observations by 1 for condition 2 or zero for condition 1 (put the result in column K).

```
Range("K2").Select
ActiveCell.FormulaR1C1 = "=RC[-9]*(RC[-8]-1)"
Selection.AutoFill Destination:=Range("K2:K" & lastrow$)
```

Double the sum of column K and subtract the sum of column B to get the difference between the condition 2 total and the condition 1 total. This goes in L2, and the absolute value goes in L3.

```
Range("L2").Select
ActiveCell.FormulaR1C1 = "=2*SUM(C[-1]:C[-1])*c*
-SUM(C[-10]:C[-10])"
Range("L3").Select
ActiveCell.FormulaR1C1 = "=ABS(R[-1]C)"
```

5 and 6. When we present the results, we quote the difference between condition means, which is the difference between totals divided by the number of blocks, in A2. The count of arrangement statistics at least as large as the actual one goes into M3, and the one-tailed probability into M4.

```
Range("M2").Select
ActiveCell.FormulaR1C1 = "=RC[-1]/R2C1"
Range("M3").Select
ActiveCell.FormulaR1C1 = "=COUNTIF(C[-4]:C[-4],""">="""&R[-1]C[-1])"
Range("M4").Select
ActiveCell.FormulaR1C1 = "=(R[-1]C+1)/(2000+1)"
```

The absolute value of the test statistic goes into M5, the count of arrangement absolute values at least as large into M6, and the two-tailed probability into M7.

```
Range("M5").Select
ActiveCell.FormulaR1C1 = "=R[-2]C[-1]/R2C1"
Range("M6").Select
ActiveCell.FormulaR1C1 = "=COUNTIF(C[-3]:C[-3],""">="""&R[-3]C[-1])"
Range("M7").SelectActiveCell.FormulaR1C1 = "=(R[-1]C+1)/(2000+1)"
End Sub
```

Small-n repeated measures design with replicates

The required file is *smallgrouprepeatedmeasureswithreps.xlsm*, containing the macro and example data (which can be seen in Table 4.7). You can replace the data in the workbook with any other suitable data, but keep the variable names the same.

Here is the column list.

A–D: Original data entered by user
E: Copy of B
F: Random numbers
G: Sum gives rearrangement difference between condition totals
H: Rearrangement test statistic
I: Stored test statistics from rearrangements
J: Absolute values of I
K: Actual difference between condition totals
L: Actual test statistic and its absolute value
M: Final results

1. As usual, we begin by clearing the columns to be used and setting up some integers. For this design, we need to know the number of observations, the number of participants, and the number of observations per participant. We have the number of participants in A2 and the number of observations per participant in A3. Multiplying these gives the number of observations.

```
Sub smallgrouprepeatedwithreps()
Columns("E:M").ClearContents
Dim j As Integer
Dim lastcase$
Dim npercase$
Dim lastobs$
lastcase = Range("A2")
npercase = Range("A3")
lastobs = lastcase * npercase
Dim lastrow$
lastrow$ = lastobs + 1
```

2. As before, we make a copy of the observations from column B into column E where they will be rearranged.

```
Range("B2:B" & lastrow$).Select
Selection.Copy
Range("E2").Select
ActiveSheet.Paste
```

3. Now set the number of rearrangements and perform the rearrangements. Rearrangements need to be within participants, so into F2 we put a random number plus the participant number from column D, and copy down the column. This means participant 1 random numbers are smaller than those for participant 2, which are smaller than for participant 3, and

so on. Thus, when we sort columns E and F on column F, the data will be rearranged within participants.

```
For j = 1 To 2000
Range("F2").Select
ActiveCell.FormulaR1C1 = "=RAND()+RC[-2]"
Selection.AutoFill Destination:=Range("F2:F" & *c*
lastrow$), Type:=xlFillDefault
Range("E2:F" & lastrow$).Select
Selection.Sort Key1:=Range("F2"), _
Order1:=xlAscending, Header:=xlGuess, _
OrderCustom:=1, MatchCase:=False, _
Orientation:=xlTopToBottom
```

Because there are only two conditions, we use the difference between condition means as the test statistic. Here is one way to obtain it. Subtract 1.5 from the condition codes in column C, and multiply the result by 2. This gives a –1 for each condition 1 and a +1 for each condition 2. Multiply these by the rearranged observations in column E, and if you sum the result, you have the difference between condition totals for the rearrangement.

```
Range("G2").Select
ActiveCell.FormulaR1C1 = "=(RC[-2]*(RC[-4]-1.5)*2)"
Selection.AutoFill Destination:=Range("G2:G" & lastrow$)
```

Now, if you divide the difference between condition totals by the number of observations and multiply the result by 2, you have the difference between condition means. This goes in H2 and is then stored at the top of column I, pushing results from previous arrangements down one row. Then proceed to the next arrangement.

```
Range("H2").Select
ActiveCell.FormulaR1C1 = "=2*SUM(C[-1])/(R2C1*R3C1)"
Selection.Copy
Range("I2").Select
Selection.Insert Shift:=xlDown
Selection.PasteSpecial Paste:=xlValues
Next
```

Because we can obtain both one- and two-tailed probabilities, we need the absolute values of the arrangement statistics. These will go into column J. We need to fill down to the last row of arrangement statistics, which will be 1 below the number of the last arrangement.

```
lastj$ = j + 1
Range("J2").Select
```

```
ActiveCell.FormulaR1C1 = "=ABS(C[-1])"
Selection.AutoFill Destination:=Range("J2:J" & lastj$)
```

4. Now we calculate the test statistic for the actual experiment in exactly the same way. K2 receives the difference between condition totals, and L2 the difference between condition means. The absolute value goes in L3.

```
Range("K2").Select
ActiveCell.FormulaR1C1 = "=(RC[-9]*(RC[-8]-1.5)*2)"
Selection.AutoFill Destination:=Range("K2:K" & lastrow$)
Range("L2").Select
ActiveCell.FormulaR1C1 = "=2*SUM(C[-1])/(R2C1*R3C1)"
Range("L3").Select
ActiveCell.FormulaR1C1 = "=ABS(R[-1]C)"
```

5 and 6. Now collect the results in column M. The actual test statistic goes into M2, and the count of arrangement statistics at least as large into M3. Divide by 2001 to get the one-tailed probability in M5.

```
Range("M2").Select
ActiveCell.FormulaR1C1 = "=RC[-1]"
Range("M3").Select
ActiveCell.FormulaR1C1 = "=COUNTIF(C[-4]:C[-4],"">=""&R[-1]C)"
Range("M4").Select
ActiveCell.FormulaR1C1 = "=(R[-1]C+1)/(2000+1)"
```

The absolute value of the actual test statistic goes in M5, the count of absolute rearrangement values at least as large into M6, and the two-tailed probability into M7.

```
Range("M5").Select
ActiveCell.FormulaR1C1 = "=R[-2]C[-1]"
Range("M6").Select
ActiveCell.FormulaR1C1 = "=COUNTIF(C[-3]:C[-3],*c*
"">=""&R[-1]C)"
Range("M7").Select
ActiveCell.FormulaR1C1 = "=(R[-1]C+1)/(2000+1)"
End Sub
```

Two-way factorial design (single-case or small-n)

The required file is *factorial.xlsm* containing the macro and data for the single-case example in sheet 1 (Table 4.8) and the small-*n* example in sheet 2 (Table 4.9). The data may be deleted and replaced with any other suitable data, but leave the variable names unchanged. Steps 2 and 3 have to be done first for factor 1, then for factor 2. Here is the column list.

A–D: Original data entered by user
E: Copy of B
F: Random numbers
G: Sum gives rearrangement difference between factor 1 level totals
H: Rearrangement test statistic for factor 1
I: Stored factor 1 test statistics from rearrangements
J: Copy of B
K: Random numbers
L: Sum gives rearrangement difference between factor 2 level totals
M: Rearrangement test statistic for factor 2
N: Stored factor 2 test statistics from rearrangements
O: Absolute values of H
P: Absolute values of M
Q: Sum gives actual difference between factor 1 level totals
R: Actual factor 1 test statistic and its absolute value
S: Sum gives actual difference between factor 2 level totals
T: Actual factor 2 test statistic and its absolute value
U: Final results

1. Begin as usual by clearing the columns to be used and setting up some integers.

```
Sub factorial()
Columns("E:U").ClearContents
Dim j As Integer
Dim lastobs$
lastobs = Range("A2")
Dim lastrow$
lastrow$ = lastobs + 1
```

To deal with factor 1, we need to have the data arranged with the factor 2 levels in blocks, so sort the columns B to D on column D.

```
Range("B2:D" & lastrow$).Select
Selection.Sort Key1:=Range("D2"), Order1:=xlAscending, _
Key2:=Range("C2"), Order2:=xlAscending, _
Header:=xlGuess, OrderCustom:=1, _
MatchCase:=False, Orientation:=xlTopToBottom
```

2. Now make a copy of the observations to column E, where they will be rearranged within levels of factor 2.

```
Range("B2:B" & lastrow$).Select
Selection.Copy
Range("E2").Select
ActiveSheet.Paste
```

3. Set the number of arrangements for factor 1. In F2, put a random number plus the factor 2 level, and copy down the column. This is so the observations at level 1 of factor 2 have smaller random numbers than those at level 2 of factor 2, and so that when we sort the copied observations using column F, they will be rearranged within levels of factor 2.

```
For j = 1 To 2000
Range("F2").Select
ActiveCell.FormulaR1C1 = "=RAND()+RC[-2]"
Selection.AutoFill Destination:=Range("F2:F" & lastrow$), _
Type:=xlFillDefault
Range("E2:F" & lastrow$).Select
Selection.Sort Key1:=Range("F2"), _
Order1:=xlAscending, Header:=xlGuess, _
OrderCustom:=1, MatchCase:=False, _
Orientation:=xlTopToBottom
```

Now we use the same device as in the last macro to get the difference between the totals of factor 1 level 2 and factor 1 level 1. Subtract 1.5 from the factor 1 levels, multiply the result by 2 (this goes in column G), then multiply the rearranged observations by column G and add. If you divide the answer by the total number of observations and multiply by 2, you have the difference between factor 1 level means. This goes in H2. Store it at the top of column I, pushing values from previous arrangements down one row. Proceed to the next arrangement within levels of factor 2.

```
Range("G2").Select
ActiveCell.FormulaR1C1 = "=(RC[-2]*(RC[-4]-1.5)*2)"
Selection.AutoFill Destination:=Range("G2:G" & *c*
lastrow$)
Range("H2").Select
ActiveCell.FormulaR1C1 = "=2*SUM(C[-1])/R2C1"
Selection.Copy
Range("I2").Select
Selection.Insert Shift:=xlDown
Selection.PasteSpecial Paste:=xlValues
Next
```

Now we start dealing with factor 2. To start with, we need to sort the data so that factor 1 levels are in blocks.

```
Range("B2:D" & lastrow$).Select
Selection.Sort Key1:=Range("C2"), Order1:=xlAscending, _
Key2:=Range("D2"), Order2:=xlAscending, _
Header:=xlGuess, OrderCustom:=1, _
MatchCase:=False, Orientation:=xlTopToBottom
```

2. Then copy the observations to rearrange within levels of factor 1.

```
Range ("B2:B" & lastrow$).Select
Selection.Copy
Range ("J2").Select
ActiveSheet.Paste
```

3. Set the number of arrangements for factor 2. In K2, put a random number plus the the factor 1 level and copy down the column. Now, when we sort the copied observations using column K, we shall get a rearrangement within levels of factor 1.

```
For j = 1 To 2000
Range ("K2").Select
ActiveCell.FormulaR1C1 = "=RAND()+RC[-8]"
Selection.AutoFill Destination:=Range ("K2:K" & lastrow$), _
Type:=xlFillDefault
Range ("J2:K" & lastrow$).Select
Selection.Sort Key1:=Range ("K2"), Order1:=xlAscending, _
Header:=xlGuess, OrderCustom:=1, MatchCase:=False, _
Orientation:=xlTopToBottom
```

Now use the same method to get the difference between the mean of factor 2 level 2 and the mean of factor 2 level 1. Store it at the top of column N, pushing values from previous arrangements down one row. Proceed to the next arrangement for factor 2.

```
Range ("L2").Select
ActiveCell.FormulaR1C1 = "=(RC[-2]*(RC[-8]-1.5)*2)"
Selection.AutoFill Destination:=Range ("L2:L" & lastrow$)
Range ("M2").Select
ActiveCell.FormulaR1C1 = "=2*SUM(C[-1])/R2C1"
Selection.Copy
Range ("N2").Select
Selection.Insert Shift:=xlDown
Selection.PasteSpecial Paste:=xlValues
Next
```

As in the previous design, we can obtain both one- and two-tailed probabilities, so we need absolute values for the test statistics. Once again, we shall need to fill down the columns of absolute values to the last row of arrangement statistics, which will be one below the number of arrangements. Column O has the absolute values for factor 1, column P for factor 2.

```
lastj$ = j+1
ActiveCell.FormulaR1C1 = "=ABS(C[-6])"
```

```
Selection.AutoFill Destination:=Range("O2:O" & lastj$)
Range("P2").Select
ActiveCell.FormulaR1C1 = "=ABS(C[-2])"
Selection.AutoFill Destination:=Range("P2:P" & lastj$)
```

4. Now we need the test statistic for the actual observations for factor 1. This goes into R2, and its absolute value into R3.

```
Range("Q2").Select
ActiveCell.FormulaR1C1 = "=(RC[-15]*(RC[-14]-1.5)*2)"
Selection.AutoFill Destination:=Range("Q2:Q" & lastrow$)
Range("R2").Select
ActiveCell.FormulaR1C1 = "=2*SUM(C[-1])/R2C1"
Range("R3").Select
ActiveCell.FormulaR1C1 = "=ABS(R[-1]C)"
```

The test statistic for the actual observations for factor 2 goes into T2, and its absolute value into T3.

```
Range("S2").Select
ActiveCell.FormulaR1C1 = "=(RC[-17]*(RC[-15]-1.5)*2)"
Selection.AutoFill Destination:=Range("S2:S" & lastrow$)
Range("T2").Select
ActiveCell.FormulaR1C1 = "=2*SUM(C[-1])/R2C1"
Range("T3").Select
ActiveCell.FormulaR1C1 = "=ABS(R[-1]C)"
```

5 and 6. Now collect all the results in column U. The factor 1 test statistic goes into U2, and the count of arrangement statistics at least large into U3. The one-tailed probability goes into U4.

```
Range("U2").Select
ActiveCell.FormulaR1C1 = "=RC[-3]"
Range("U3").Select
ActiveCell.FormulaR1C1 = "=COUNTIF(C[-12]:C[-12],""">="""&R[-1]C)"
Range("U4").Select
ActiveCell.FormulaR1C1 = "=(R[-1]C+1)/(2000+1)"
```

The absolute value of the test statistic for factor 1 goes into U5, and the count of absolute values of arrangements statistics at least as large goes into U6, with the two-tailed probability in U7.

```
Range("U5").Select
ActiveCell.FormulaR1C1 = "=R[-2]C[-3]"
Range("U6").Select
ActiveCell.FormulaR1C1 = "=COUNTIF(C[-6]:C[-6],""">="""&R[-1]C)"
Range("U7").Select
ActiveCell.FormulaR1C1 = "=(R[-1]C+1)/(2000+1)"
```

The results for factor 2 follow in exactly the same way from U8 to U13.

```
Range("U8").Select
ActiveCell.FormulaR1C1 = "=R[-6]C[-1]"
Range("U9").Select
ActiveCell.FormulaR1C1 = "=COUNTIF(C[-7]:C[-7],""">="""&R[-1]C)"
Range("U10").Select
ActiveCell.FormulaR1C1 = "=(R[-1]C+1)/(2000+1)"
Range("U11").Select
ActiveCell.FormulaR1C1 = "=R[-8]C[-1]"
Range("U12").Select
ActiveCell.FormulaR1C1 = "=COUNTIF(C[-5]:C[-5],""">="""&R[-1]C)"
Range("U13").Select
ActiveCell.FormulaR1C1 = "=(R[-1]C+1)/(2000+1)"
End Sub
```

Single-case AB design

The macro and example data (which can be seen in Table 4.10) are in *singlecaseAB.xlsm*. The data may be replaced by the user's own or any other suitable example, but keep the variable names the same. If a one-tailed test is to be used, the alternative hypothesis must be that the intervention increases the mean score. If this is not the case, subtract all observations from a convenient round number that is larger than any observation. Here is the column list.

A–C: Original data entered by user
D: ID numbers
E: Cumulative probabilities for intervention points
F: List of intervention points
G: Random number
H: Random intervention point from lookup table (columns E–F)
I: Phase codes for random intervention point
J: Baseline and intervention totals and counts for random intervention
K: Test statistics for this random intervention
L: Stored test statistics from random interventions
M: Absolute values of L
N: Baseline and intervention totals and counts for actual intervention
O: Final results

1. We begin as usual by clearing the columns to be used.

```
Sub singlecaseAB()
Columns("D:O").ClearContents
```

Now we calculate the observation number for the last possible intervention point, which is the total number of observations minus the minimum number for the intervention phase plus 1. This goes into A5.

```
Range("A5").Select
ActiveCell.FormulaR1C1 = "=R2C1 - R4C1 + 1"
```

Now calculate the number of possible intervention points, which is the number of the last possible one minus the minimum number for the baseline phase. This goes into A6.

```
Range("A6").Select
ActiveCell.FormulaR1C1 = "=R5C1 - R3C1"
```

Set up some integers as in previous macros. As well as a counter for rearrangements and the row number for the last observation and its phase code (lastrow), we shall need the row number for the bottom of columns of random intervention points (lastperm).

```
Dim j As Integer
Dim last_i As Integer
last_i = Range("A2")
Dim lastrow$
lastrow$ = last_i + 1
Dim lastperm$
lastperm$ = Range("A6") + 1
```

2. We shall need to number the observations from 1 to the total number. We put these identification numbers in column D.

```
Range("D2").Select
ActiveCell.FormulaR1C1 = "1"
Range("D3").Select
ActiveCell.FormulaR1C1 = "2"
Range("D2:D3").Select
Selection.AutoFill Destination:=Range("D2:D" & lastrow$), _
Type:=xlFillDefault
```

We shall need the cumulative probabilities for the possible intervention points, which will make the first column of a lookup table. To get the cumulative probabilities, we need to increase in A5 (the number of possible intervention points) equal steps from zero.

```
Range("E2").Select
ActiveCell.FormulaR1C1 = "=(RC[-1]-1)/R6C1"
```

```
Selection.AutoFill Destination:=Range("E2:E" & lastperm$), _
Type:=xlFillDefault
```

In column F, we list the possible intervention points. This will be the second column of the lookup table.

```
Range("F2").Select
ActiveCell.FormulaR1C1 = "=RC[-2]+R3C1"
Selection.AutoFill Destination:=Range("F2:F" & lastperm$), _
Type:=xlFillDefault
Columns("E:F").Select
ActiveWorkbook.Names.Add Name:="lookup", RefersToR1C1:="=C5:C6"
```

3. Now we set the number of arrangements. For the phase designs, an arrangement is a choice of intervention point. Put a random number into G2.

```
For j = 1 To 2000
Range("G2").Select
ActiveCell.FormulaR1C1 = "=RAND()"
```

Now we use the lookup table to get the randomly chosen intervention point. The random number in G2 will be compared with the first column (E) of the lookup table to find the largest number that is smaller than G2. Then the column F number from the same row will be put in H2. This is the intervention point corresponding to the random number in G2.

```
Range("H2").Select
ActiveCell.FormulaR1C1 = *c*
"=VLOOKUP(RC[-1],lookup,2)"
```

Now we need a column with 0s until the intervention point and 1s from the intervention point to the last row of data. This is where we use column D, which numbers the observations from one.

```
Range("I2").Select
ActiveCell.FormulaR1C1 = "=IF(R2C8>RC[-5],0,1)"
Selection.AutoFill Destination:=Range("I2:I" & lastrow$), _
Type:=xlFillDefault
```

Now we have to sum the observations from intervention (J2) and before intervention (J3).

```
Range("J2").Select
ActiveCell.FormulaR1C1 = _
"=SUMIF(C[-1]:C[-1],"">0"",C[-8]:C[-8])"
Range("J3").Select
```

```
ActiveCell.FormulaR1C1 = _
"=SUMIF(C[-1]:C[-1],""=0"",C[-8]:C[-8])"
```

We also need the number of observations from intervention (J4) and the number before intervention (J5).

```
Range("J4").Select
ActiveCell.FormulaR1C1 = *c*
"=R[-2]C[-9] - R[-2]C[-2] + 1"
Range("J5").Select
ActiveCell.FormulaR1C1 = "=R[-3]C[-2]-1"
```

The test statistic is the intervention mean minus the baseline mean. This is calculated in K2 and stored at the top of column L, pushing values from previous arrangements down one row. Move to the next arrangement.

```
Range("K2").Select
ActiveCell.FormulaR1C1 = *c*
"=RC[-1]/R[2]C[-1]-R[1]C[-1]/R[3]C[-1]"
Selection.Copy
Range("L2").SelectSelection.Insert Shift:=xlDown
Selection.PasteSpecial Paste:=xlValues
Next
```

Because both one- and two-tailed probabilities may be calculated, we need the absolute values of the arrangement test statistics. They go into column M.

```
lastj$ = j+1
Range("M2").Select
ActiveCell.FormulaR1C1 = "=ABS(C[-1])"
Selection.AutoFill Destination:=Range("M2:M" & lastj$), _
Type:=xlFillDefault
```

4. Now we need the test statistic from the actual experiment. The sum of intervention observations goes into N2, and the baseline sum into N3.

```
Range("N2").Select
ActiveCell.FormulaR1C1 = _
"=SUMIF(C[-11]:C[-11],"">0"",C[-12]:C[-12])"
Range("N3").Select
ActiveCell.FormulaR1C1 = _
"=SUMIF(C[-11]:C[-11],""=0"",C[-12]:C[-12])"
```

The count of observations from intervention goes into N4, and the baseline count into N5.

```
Range ("N4") .Select
ActiveCell.FormulaR1C1 = _
"=COUNTIF(C[-11]:C[-11],"">0"")"
Range ("N5") .Select
ActiveCell.FormulaR1C1 = _
"=COUNTIF(C[-11]:C[-11],""=0"")"
```

5 and 6. The test statistic is the intervention mean minus the baseline mean and goes into O2. The count of arrangement statistics at least as large goes into O3, and the one-tailed probability into O4.

```
Range ("O2") .Select
ActiveCell.FormulaR1C1 = *c*
"=RC[-1]/R[2]C[-1]-R[1]C[-1]/R[3]C[-1]"
Range ("O3") .Select
ActiveCell.FormulaR1C1 = _
"=COUNTIF(C[-3]:C[-3],"">=""&R[-1]C)"
Range ("O4") .Select
ActiveCell.FormulaR1C1 = "=(R[-1]C+1)/(2000+1)"
```

The absolute value of the test statistic, the count of arrangement values at least as large, and the two-tailed probability go into O5, O6, and O7, respectively.

```
Range ("O5") .Select
ActiveCell.FormulaR1C1 = "=ABS(R[-3]C)"
Range ("O6") .Select
ActiveCell.FormulaR1C1 = _
"=COUNTIF(C[-2]:C[-2],"">=""&R[-1]C)"
Range ("O7") .Select
ActiveCell.FormulaR1C1 = "=(R[-1]C+1)/(2000+1)"
End Sub
```

Single-case ABA design

The macro and example data (which may be seen in Table 4.12) are in *singlecaseABA.xlsm*. The data may be replaced by the user's own or any other suitable example, but keep the variable names the same. If a one-tailed test is to be used, the alternative hypothesis must be that the intervention increases the mean score. If this is not the case, subtract all observations from a convenient round number that is larger than any observation. Here is the column list.

A–C: Original data entered by user
D: ID numbers for possible intervention and withdrawal pairs

E–F: Preliminary lists to get intervention and withdrawal pairs

G: Cumulative probabilities for intervention and withdrawal pairs

H–I: List of intervention (H) and withdrawal (I) pairs

J: Random number

K: Random intervention and withdrawal from lookup table (columns G–I)

L: Phase codes for random intervention and withdrawal

M: Baseline–withdrawal and intervention totals and counts for random intervention and withdrawal

N: Test statistic for random intervention and withdrawal

O: Stored test statistics for random intervention and withdrawal pairs

P: Absolute values of O

Q: Baseline–withdrawal and intervention totals and counts for actual intervention and withdrawal

R: Final results

1. We begin as for the AB design, but this time we need the number of possible intervention points (A6) and also the number of possible intervention and withdrawal pairs (A7).

```
Sub singlecaseABA()
Columns("D:S").ClearContents
Range("A6").Select
ActiveCell.FormulaR1C1 = "=(R2C1-R3C1-R4C1-R5C1+1)"
Range("A7").Select
ActiveCell.FormulaR1C1 = "=R6C1*(R6C1+1)/2"
```

Now set up integers to count arrangements, and denote the last row of data (lastrow) and the last row of the list of intervention and withdrawal pairs (lastperm).

```
Dim last_i As Integer
last_i = Range("A2")
Dim lastrow$
lastrow$ = last_i + 1
Dim lastperm$
lastperm$ = Range("A7") + 1
```

2. We shall need to number a list of the possible intervention and withdrawal pairs. Column D contains the numbers 1, 2, ... up to lastperm.

```
Range("D2").Select
ActiveCell.FormulaR1C1 = "1"
Range("D3").Select
ActiveCell.FormulaR1C1 = "2"
Range("D2:D3").Select
```

```
Selection.AutoFill Destination:=Range("D2:D" & lastperm$), _
Type:=xlFillDefault
```

If the last possible intervention point is used, there is only one possible withdrawal point; if the penultimate possible intervention point is used, there are two possible withdrawal points; if the third-to-last intervention point is used, there are three possible withdrawal points; and so on. We shall need a list of possible pairs of intervention and withdrawal points, and because of the pattern just noted, a first step will be to make a list of the numbers 1, 2, 2, 3, 3, 3, 4, 4, 4, 4, 5.... You need some knowledge of sequences and series to see how this can be achieved, but you can check that the formula in E2 does work. Note that the function INT takes the integer part, so INT(5.2) = 5 but also INT(5.8) = 5.

```
Range("E2").Select
ActiveCell.FormulaR1C1 = "=INT(0.5+SQRT(2*RC[-1]))"
Selection.AutoFill Destination:=Range("E2:E" & lastperm$), _
Type:=xlFillDefault
```

The next step to providing the list of intervention and withdrawal pairs is to list the numbers 1, 1, 2, 1, 2, 3, 1, 2, 3, 4, 1.... Again, you can check that this is what goes into column F. Into column G goes a list of cumulative probabilities for the intervention withdrawal pairs.

```
Range("F2").Select
ActiveCell.FormulaR1C1 = *c*
"=RC[-2]-RC[-1]*(RC[-1]-1)/2"
Selection.AutoFill Destination:=Range("F2:F" & lastperm$), _
Type:=xlFillDefault
Range("G2").Select
ActiveCell.FormulaR1C1 = "=(RC[-3]-1)/R7C1"
Selection.AutoFill Destination:=Range("G2:G" & lastperm$), _
Type:=xlFillDefault
```

Now we list the intervention points (from last to first) in column H and the corresponding withdrawal points in column I. Columns E and F enable us to do this. After running the macro, it's easy to check that they are correct. Columns G to I become our lookup table.

```
Range("H2").Select
ActiveCell.FormulaR1C1 = "=R2C1-R4C1-R5C1+2-RC[-3]"
Selection.AutoFill Destination:=Range("H2:H" & lastperm$), _
Type:=xlFillDefault
Range("I2").Select
ActiveCell.FormulaR1C1 = "=R2C1-R5C1+2-RC[-3]"
Selection.AutoFill Destination:=Range("I2:I" & lastperm$), _
```

```
Type:=xlFillDefault
Columns("G:I").Select
ActiveWorkbook.Names.Add Name:="lookup", RefersToR1C1:="=C7:C9"
```

3. Now we are ready to do the rearrangements. Here a rearrangement is a choice of intervention and withdrawal pair. Into J2 we put a random number. In the lookup table, compare this with the cumulative probabilities and read off the intervention and withdrawal points into K2 and K3 from the correct row of columns H and I.

```
For j = 1 To 2000
Range("J2").Select
ActiveCell.FormulaR1C1 = "=RAND()"
Range("K2").Select
ActiveCell.FormulaR1C1 = "=VLOOKUP(RC[-1],lookup,2)"
Range("K3").Select
ActiveCell.FormulaR1C1 = "=VLOOKUP(R[-1]C[-1],lookup,3)"
```

Now into column L, we put a column of 0s and 1s to indicate the correct phase according to the randomly chosen pair of intervention and withdrawal points in K2 and K3. For this, we use the numbers assigned to the intervention withdrawal pairs in column D.

```
Range("L2").Select
ActiveCell.FormulaR1C1 = _
"=IF(RC[-8]<R2C11,0,IF(RC[-8]>=R3C11,0,1))"
Selection.AutoFill Destination:=Range("L2:L" & lastrow$), _
Type:=xlFillDefault
```

Now we find the test statistic, the intervention mean minus the mean of baseline and withdrawal phases. This is done as in the previous macro. The result is stored at the top of column O, previous values being pushed down one row. Then proceed to the next arrangement.

```
Range("M2").Select
ActiveCell.FormulaR1C1 = _
"=SUMIF(C[-1]:C[-1],"">0"",C[-11]:C[-11])"
Range("M3").Select
ActiveCell.FormulaR1C1 = _
"=SUMIF(C[-1]:C[-1],""=0"",C[-11]:C[-11])"
Range("M4").Select
ActiveCell.FormulaR1C1 = "=COUNTIF(C[-1]:C[-1],"">0"")"
Range("M5").Select
ActiveCell.FormulaR1C1 = _
"=COUNTIF(C[-1]:C[-1],""=0"")"
Range("N2").Select
ActiveCell.FormulaR1C1 = "=RC[-1]/R[2]C[-1]-R[1]C[-1]/R[3]C[-1]"
Selection.Copy
```

```
Range("O2").Select
Selection.Insert Shift:=xlDown
Selection.PasteSpecial Paste:=xlValues
Next
```

Because both one- and two-tailed probabilities may be calculated, we need the absolute values of the test statistics. They go into column P.

```
lastj$ = j + 1
Range("P2").Select
ActiveCell.FormulaR1C1 = "=ABS(C[-1])"
Selection.AutoFill Destination:=Range("P2:P" & lastj$), _
Type:=xlFillDefault
```

4. Now we need the test statistic for the actual data, calculated in the same way.

```
Range("Q2").Select
ActiveCell.FormulaR1C1 = _
"=SUMIF(C[-14]:C[-14],"">0"",C[-15]:C[-15])"
Range("Q3").Select
ActiveCell.FormulaR1C1 = _
"=SUMIF(C[-14]:C[-14],""=0"",C[-15]:C[-15])"
Range("Q4").Select
ActiveCell.FormulaR1C1 = _
"=COUNTIF(C[-14]:C[-14],"">0"")"
Range("Q5").Select
ActiveCell.FormulaR1C1 = _
"=COUNTIF(C[-14]:C[-14],""=0"")"
Range("R2").Select
ActiveCell.FormulaR1C1 = *c*
"=RC[-1]/R[2]C[-1]-R[1]C[-1]/R[3]C[-1]"
```

5 and 6. Now we count arrangement statistics at least as large as the actual one and divide by 2001 to get the one-tailed probability. The absolute value of the actual test statistic goes into R5, the count of absolute arrangement statistics at least as large goes into R6, and the two-tailed probability goes into R7.

```
Range("R3").Select
ActiveCell.FormulaR1C1 = "=COUNTIF(C[-3]:C[-3],"">=""&R[-1]C)"
Range("R4").Select
ActiveCell.FormulaR1C1 = "=(R[-1]C+1)/(2000+1)"
Range("R5").Select
ActiveCell.FormulaR1C1 = "=ABS(R[-3]C)"
Range("R6").Select
ActiveCell.FormulaR1C1 = "=COUNTIF(C[-2]:C[-2],"">=""&R[-1]C)"
Range("R7").Select
ActiveCell.FormulaR1C1 = "=(R[-1]C+1)/(2000+1)"
End Sub
```

Multiple baseline AB design

The macro and example data (which may be seen in Table 4.13) are in *multiplebaselineAB.xlsm*. The data may be replaced by the user's own or any other suitable example, but the ranges must also be edited for the names DATA and LEVEL. Also, keep the variable names the same. In the **Name Manager** dialog box, replace 31 (the last row of example data) by the last row of the new data.

If a one-tailed test is to be used, the alternative hypotheses must be that the interventions increase the mean scores. If the alternative hypotheses predict a decrease, subtract all observations from a convenient round number that is larger than any observation. Here is the column list.

A–D: Original data entered by user
E: A code that combines phase and participant (changed for each arrangement)
F: ID numbers
G: Cumulative probabilities for intervention points
H: List of intervention points
I: Random number
J: Random intervention point for one participant from lookup table (columns G–H)
K: Phase codes for random intervention for one participant
L: Phase codes for random intervention points for all participants for this arrangement
M: A column to assist calculating the test statistic for this arrangement
N: Phase means for each participant
O: Multiply columns M and N
P: Sum column O (test statistic for this arrangement)
Q: Stored arrangement test statistics
R: Absolute values of Q
S: Actual test statistic and final results

1. We begin as usual by clearing the area to be used. This time we set up integers to count both arrangements (j) and participants (s). We calculate the last possible intervention point (A6) and the number of possible intervention points (A7 for each participant). The number of participants is read from A2, and the number of observations per participant from A3. The last row of data is calculated from these. The last row for a list of possible intervention points (for each participant) is one more than the number of arrangements. We also need the row number of the bottom of the column of phase codes for each randomly assigned intervention (lastphase).

```
Sub multiplebaselineAB()
Columns("F:R").ClearContents
Dim j As Integer
Dim s As Integer
Range("A6").Select
ActiveCell.FormulaR1C1 = "=R3C1 - R5C1 + 1"
Range("A7").Select
ActiveCell.FormulaR1C1 = "=R6C1 - R4C1"
Dim lastsubject As Integer
lastsubject = Range("A2")
Dim last_i As Integer
last_i = Range("A3")
Dim lastrow$
lastrow$ = lastsubject * last_i + 1
Dim lastperm$
lastperm$ = Range("A7") + 1
Dim lastphase$
lastphase$ = last_i + 1
```

2. In column F, we number the observations from 1 to the last observation on the last participant.

```
Range("F2").Select
ActiveCell.FormulaR1C1 = "1"
Range("F3").Select
ActiveCell.FormulaR1C1 = "2"
Range("F2:F3").Select
Selection.AutoFill Destination:=Range("F2:F" & lastrow$), _
Type:=xlFillDefault
```

Into column G, put the cumulative probabilities for the possible intervention points.

```
Range("G2").Select
ActiveCell.FormulaR1C1 = "=(RC[-1]-1)/R7C1"
Selection.AutoFill Destination:=Range("G2:G" & lastperm$), _
Type:=xlFillDefault
```

In column H, list the possible intervention points, then make a lookup table from columns G and H.

```
Range("H2").Select
ActiveCell.FormulaR1C1 = "=RC[-2]+R4C1"
Selection.AutoFill Destination:=Range("H2:H" & lastperm$), _
Type:=xlFillDefault
Columns("G:H").Select
ActiveWorkbook.Names.Add Name:="lookup", RefersToR1C1:="=C7:C8"
```

3. Now start the rearrangements (for this design, a rearrangement is a choice of intervention point for each participant). Column L will store the

phase codes for all participants at each arrangement, so it is cleared at the start of each arrangement so that they are not accumulated for all arrangements. For each arrangement, we have to work through the participants one at a time; and for each one, we put a random number in I2.

```
For j = 1 To 2000
Columns("L").ClearContents
For s = 1 To lastsubject
Range("I2").Select
ActiveCell.FormulaR1C1 = "=RAND()"
```

Use the random number to find the intervention point for this participant from the lookup table. It goes in J2, then a column of 0s and 1s for the corresponding phases goes in column K.

```
Range("J2").Select
ActiveCell.FormulaR1C1 = "=VLOOKUP(RC[-1],lookup,2)"
Range("K2").Select
ActiveCell.FormulaR1C1 = "=IF(R2C10>RC[-5],0,1)"
Selection.AutoFill Destination:=Range("K2:K" & lastphase$), _
Type:=xlFillDefault
```

Store this set of phase codes in the top of column L, pushing down the set from the previous participant. Then move to the next participant.

```
Range("K2:K" & lastphase$).Select
Selection.Copy
Range("L2").Select
Selection.Insert Shift:=xlDown
Selection.PasteSpecial Paste:=xlValues
Next
```

When we have stepped through all participants, column L will contain phase codes for all participants according to the randomly chosen intervention points for the current arrangement. We need to find the difference between phase means for each participant, and then add the results over participants. This is not the same as finding the difference between the overall intervention mean and the overall baseline mean. As a first step, make a column with a −1 in the row corresponding to the start of baseline and a +1 at the start of intervention for each participant. All other values in the column will be zero. Start M2 off at −1, but from M3 down all you need do is go to column L and from each row subtract the row above.

```
Range("M2").Select
ActiveCell.FormulaR1C1 = -1
```

```
Range("M3").Select
ActiveCell.FormulaR1C1 = "=RC[-1]-R[-1]C[-1]"
Selection.AutoFill Destination:=Range("M3:M" & lastrow$), _
Type:=xlFillDefault
```

Now we need a code that combines phase and participant. This goes in column E. This column of codes has the name "level."

```
Range("E2").Select
ActiveCell.FormulaR1C1 = "=10*RC[-1]+RC[7]"
Selection.AutoFill Destination:=Range("E2:E" & lastrow$), _
Type:=xlFillDefault
```

We use this new code to obtain phase means for each participant. They fill up column N.

```
Range("N2").Select
ActiveCell.FormulaR1C1 = *c*
"=SUMIF(level,C5,data)/COUNTIF(level,C5)"
Selection.AutoFill Destination:=Range("N2:N" & lastrow$), _
Type:=xlFillDefault
```

Now multiply by the column with a −1 at the start of each baseline, a +1 at the start of each intervention, and zeros elsewhere. Summing this column (into P2) gives the test statistic for this arrangement.

```
Range("O2").Select
ActiveCell.FormulaR1C1 = "=RC[-1]*RC[-2]"
Selection.AutoFill Destination:=Range("O2:O" & lastrow$), _
Type:=xlFillDefault
Range("P2").Select
ActiveCell.FormulaR1C1 = "=SUM(C[-1])"
```

Store at the top of column Q, pushing values from previous arrangements down one row. Then go to the next arrangement.

```
Selection.Copy
Range("Q2").Select
Selection.Insert Shift:=xlDown
Selection.PasteSpecial Paste:=xlValues
Next
```

Note the last row of arrangement statistics because we shall want to make a column of absolute values.

```
lastj$ = j + 1
```

4. But first get the test statistic for the actual data in the same way as we used for the arrangement statistics. The final sum (into S2) is done after we fill column R with the absolute values of the arrangement statistics.

```
Range ("M2") .Select
ActiveCell.FormulaR1C1 = -1
Range ("M3") .Select
ActiveCell.FormulaR1C1 = "=RC[-10]-R[-1]C[-10]"
Selection.AutoFill Destination:=Range("M3:M" & lastrow$), _
Type:=xlFillDefault
Range ("E2") .Select
ActiveCell.FormulaR1C1 = "=10*RC[-1]+RC[-2]"
Selection.AutoFill Destination:=Range("E2:E" & lastrow$), _
Type:=xlFillDefault
Range ("N2") .Select
ActiveCell.FormulaR1C1 = *c*
"=SUMIF(level,C5,data)/COUNTIF(level,C5)"
Selection.AutoFill Destination:=Range("N2:N" & lastrow$), _
Type:=xlFillDefault
Range ("O2") .Select
ActiveCell.FormulaR1C1 = "=RC[-1]*RC[-2]"
Selection.AutoFill Destination:=Range("O2:O" & lastrow$), _
Type:=xlFillDefault
```

5 and 6. Put the absolute values of the arrangement statistics into column R, then collect results in column S. S2 has the actual test statistic, S3 the count of arrangement statistics at least as large, and S4 the one-tailed probability. S5 has the absolute value of the actual test statistic, S6 the count of absolute values of arrangement statistics at least as large, and S7 the two-tailed probability.

```
Range ("R2") .Select
ActiveCell.FormulaR1C1 = "=ABS(C[-1])"
Selection.AutoFill Destination:=Range("R2:R" & lastj$), _
Type:=xlFillDefault
Range ("S2") .Select
ActiveCell.FormulaR1C1 = "=SUM(C[-4])"
Range ("S3") .Select
ActiveCell.FormulaR1C1 = "=COUNTIF(C[-2]:C[-2],""">=""&R[-1]C)"
Range ("S4") .Select
ActiveCell.FormulaR1C1 = "=(R[-1]C+1)/(2000+1)"
Range ("S5") .Select
ActiveCell.FormulaR1C1 = "=ABS(R[-3]C)"
Range ("S6") .Select
ActiveCell.FormulaR1C1 = "=COUNTIF(C[-1]:C[-1],""">=""&R[-1]C)"
Range ("S7") .Select
ActiveCell.FormulaR1C1 = "=(R[-1]C+1)/(2000+1)
End Sub
```

Multiple baseline ABA design

The macro and example data (which may be seen in Table 4.14) are in *multiplebaselineABA.xlsm*. The data may be replaced by the user's own or any other suitable example, but the ranges must also be edited for the names DATA and LEVEL. In the **Name Manager** dialog box, replace 31 (the last row of example data) by the last row of the new data. Keep the variable names the same.

If a one-tailed test is to be used, the alternative hypothesis must be that the intervention increases the mean scores. If the alternative hypothesis predicts a decrease, subtract all observations from a convenient round number that is larger than any observation. Here is the column list.

A–D: Original data entered by user
E: A code combining phase and participant (changed for each arrangement)
F: ID numbers for possible intervention and withdrawal pairs
G–H: Preliminary lists to get intervention and withdrawal pairs
I: Cumulative probabilities for intervention and withdrawal pairs
J–K: List of intervention (J) and withdrawal (K) pairs
L: Random number
M: Random intervention and withdrawal from lookup table (columns I–K) for one participant
N: Phase codes for random intervention and withdrawal for one participant
O: Phase codes for random intervention and withdrawal for all participants for this arrangement
P: A column to assist calculating the test statistic for this arrangement
Q: Phase means for each participant
R: Multiply columns P and Q
S: Sum column R (test statistic for this arrangement)
T: Stored arrangement test statistics
U: Absolute value of T
V: Actual test statistics and final results

1. We begin as in the previous macro, but this time the number of possible intervention withdrawal pairs for each participant is in A8.

```
Columns("F:V").ClearContents
Dim j As Integer
Dim s As Integer
Range("A7").Select
ActiveCell.FormulaR1C1 = "=(R3C1-R4C1-R5C1-R6C1+1)"
```

```
Range("A8").Select
ActiveCell.FormulaR1C1 = "=R7C1*(R7C1+1)/2"
Dim lastsubject As Integer
lastsubject = Range("A2")
Dim last_i As Integer
last_i = Range("A3")
Dim lastrow$
lastrow$ = lastsubject * last_i + 1
Dim lastperm$
lastperm$ = Range("A8") + 1
Dim lastphase$
lastphase$ = last_i + 1
```

2. Now we have to list the possible intervention–withdrawal pairs. The method is the same as that used in the single-case ABA design. The pairs go into columns J and K. Into column I go the cumulative probabilities, so that columns I to K form the lookup table.

```
Range("F2").Select
ActiveCell.FormulaR1C1 = "1"
Range("F3").Select
ActiveCell.FormulaR1C1 = "2"
Range("F2:F3").Select
Selection.AutoFill Destination:=Range("F2:F" & lastphase$), _
Type:=xlFillDefault
Range("G2").Select
ActiveCell.FormulaR1C1 = "=INT(0.5+SQRT(2*RC[-1]))"
Selection.AutoFill Destination:=Range("G2:G" & lastperm$), _
Type:=xlFillDefault
Range("H2").Select
ActiveCell.FormulaR1C1 = "=RC[-2]-RC[-1]*(RC[-1]-1)/2"
Selection.AutoFill Destination:=Range("H2:H" & lastperm$), _
Type:=xlFillDefault
Range("J2").Select
ActiveCell.FormulaR1C1 = "=R3C1-R5C1-R6C1+2-RC[-3]"
Selection.AutoFill Destination:=Range("J2:J" & lastperm$), _
Type:=xlFillDefault
Range("K2").Select
ActiveCell.FormulaR1C1 = "=R3C1-R6C1+2-RC[-3]"
Selection.AutoFill Destination:=Range("K2:K" & lastperm$), _
Type:=xlFillDefault
Range("I2").Select
ActiveCell.FormulaR1C1 = "=(RC[-3]-1)/R8C1"
Selection.AutoFill Destination:=Range("I2:I" & lastperm$), _
Type:=xlFillDefault
Columns("I:K").Select
ActiveWorkbook.Names.Add Name:="lookup", RefersToR1C1:="=C9:C11"
```

3. Now we are ready to do the arrangements (for this design, an arrangement is a choice of intervention–withdrawal pair for each participant). For each arrangement, column O will store the phase codes for the participants,

so it is cleared at the start of each arrangement. For each subject, a random number is put into L2, and the lookup table is used to find the corresponding intervention–withdrawal pair, which go into M2 and M3. Column N is used for the corresponding phase codes, and these are then stored at the top of column O, pushing down the codes for the previous participant. Then we move to the next participant.

```
For j = 1 To 2000
Columns("O").ClearContents
For s = 1 To lastsubject
Range("L2").Select
ActiveCell.FormulaR1C1 = "=RAND()"
Range("M2").Select
ActiveCell.FormulaR1C1 = "=VLOOKUP(RC[-1],lookup,2)"
Range("M3").Select
ActiveCell.FormulaR1C1 = "=VLOOKUP(R[-1]C[-1],lookup,3)"
Range("N2").Select
ActiveCell.FormulaR1C1 = *c*
"=IF(RC[-8]<R2C13,0,IF(RC[-8]>=R3C13,0,1))"
Selection.AutoFill Destination:=Range("N2:N" & lastphase$), _
Type:=xlFillDefault
Range("N2:N" & lastphase$).Select
Selection.Copy
Range("O2").Select
Selection.Insert Shift:=xlDown
Selection.PasteSpecial Paste:=xlValues
Next
```

Once we have the phase codes for all participants for this arrangement, we find the test statistic. We need the intervention mean minus the mean for baseline and withdrawal for each participant. The test statistic is the sum over participants. We use the same method as for the multiple baseline AB design. Store the test statistic at the top of column T, pushing previous values down one row, and move to the next arrangement.

```
Range("P2").Select
ActiveCell.FormulaR1C1 = 0
Range("P3").Select
ActiveCell.FormulaR1C1 = "=RC[-1]-R[-1]C[-1]"
Selection.AutoFill Destination:=Range("P3:P" & lastrow$), _
Type:=xlFillDefault
Range("E2").Select
ActiveCell.FormulaR1C1 = "=10*RC[-1]+RC[10]"
Selection.AutoFill Destination:=Range("E2:E" & lastrow$), _
Type:=xlFillDefault
Range("Q2").Select
ActiveCell.FormulaR1C1 = *c*
"=SUMIF(level,C5,data)/COUNTIF(level,C5)"
Selection.AutoFill Destination:=Range("Q2:Q" & lastrow$), _
```

```
Type:=xlFillDefault
Range("R2").Select
ActiveCell.FormulaR1C1 = "=RC[-1]*RC[-2]"
Selection.AutoFill Destination:=Range("R2:R" & lastrow$), _
Type:=xlFillDefault
Range("S2").Select
ActiveCell.FormulaR1C1 = "=SUM(C[-1])"
Selection.Copy
Range("T2").Select
Selection.Insert Shift:=xlDown
Selection.PasteSpecial Paste:=xlValues
Next
```

4. Now we need the test statistic for the actual experiment, but because we shall need absolute values for a two-tailed probability, we first note the row number of the last arrangement statistic.

```
lastj$ = j + 1
Range("P2").Select
ActiveCell.FormulaR1C1 = 0
Range("P3").Select
ActiveCell.FormulaR1C1 = "=RC[-13]-R[-1]C[-13]"
Selection.AutoFill Destination:=Range("P3:P" & lastrow$), _
Type:=xlFillDefault
Range("E2").Select
ActiveCell.FormulaR1C1 =
"=10*RC[-1]+RC[-2]"
Selection.AutoFill Destination:=Range("E2:E" & lastrow$), _
Type:=xlFillDefault
Range("Q2").Select
ActiveCell.FormulaR1C1 = "=SUMIF(level,C5,data)/COUNTIF(level,C5)"
Selection.AutoFill Destination:=Range("Q2:Q" & lastrow$), _
Type:=xlFillDefault
Range("R2").Select
ActiveCell.FormulaR1C1 = "=RC[-1]*RC[-2]"
Selection.AutoFill Destination:=Range("R2:R" & lastrow$), _
Type:=xlFillDefault
```

Column U receives the absolute values of the arrangement test statistics.

```
Range("U2").Select
ActiveCell.FormulaR1C1 = "=ABS(C[-1])"
Selection.AutoFill Destination:=Range("U2:U" & lastj$), _
Type:=xlFillDefault
```

5 and 6. The results are collected in column V. The actual test statistic, count of arrangement statistics at least as large, and one-tailed probability are in V2, V3, and V4. V5 to V7 contain the absolute value of the actual test statistic, the count of absolute values of the arrangement statistics at least as large, and the two-tailed probability.

```
Range("V2").Select
ActiveCell.FormulaR1C1 = "=SUM(C[-4])"
Range("V3").Select
ActiveCell.FormulaR1C1 = "=COUNTIF(C[-2]:C[-2],""">=""&R[-1]C)"
Range("V4").Select
ActiveCell.FormulaR1C1 = "=(R[-1]C+1)/(2000+1)"
Range("V5").Select
ActiveCell.FormulaR1C1 = "=ABS(R[-3]C)"
Range("V6").Select
ActiveCell.FormulaR1C1 = "=COUNTIF(C[-1]:C[-1],""">=""&R[-1]C)"
Range("V7").Select
ActiveCell.FormulaR1C1 = "=(R[-1]C+1)/(2000+1)"
End Sub
```

Design to test ordinal predictions

The macro and example data (which may be seen in Table 4.15) are in
ordereffects.xlsm. The data may be replaced by the user's own or any suitable example, but variable names must be retained. The coding should
make the predicted correlation positive. Here is the column list.

A–C: Original data entered by user
D: Copy of B
E: Random numbers
F: Multiply columns D and C
G: Rearrangement test statistic (sum of column F)
H: Stored test statistics from all rearrangements
I: Multiply columns B and C
J: Actual test statistic (sum of I) and final results

1 and 2. As usual, we begin by clearing the area to be used and setting up
some integers. This time we only need a counter for arrangements (j) and
the last row of data. Then we copy the observations in column B to column
D, where they will be rearranged.

```
Sub ordereffects()
Columns("D:J").ClearContents
Dim j As Integer
Dim lastsubject As Integer
lastsubject = Range("A2")
Dim lastrow$
lastrow$ = lastsubject + 1
Range("B2:B" & lastrow$).Select
Selection.Copy
Range("D2").Select
ActiveSheet.Paste
```

3. Now we do the rearrangements. Put a column of random numbers in column E, and then sort columns D and E on column E, so we get a rearrangement of the copied observations in column D.

```
For j = 1 To 2000
Range("E2").Select
ActiveCell.FormulaR1C1 = "=Rand()"
Selection.AutoFill Destination:=Range("E2:E" & lastrow$), _
Type:=xlFillDefault
Range("D2:E" & lastrow$).Select
Selection.Sort Key1:=Range("E2"), Order1:=xlAscending, _
Header:=xlGuess, OrderCustom:=1, MatchCase:=False, _
Orientation:=xlTopToBottom
```

The test statistic is the sum of products of the observations and their predicted order. For this arrangement, the products go into column F and the sum into G2. This is stored at the top of column H, pushing previous values down one row. Then move to the next arrangement.

```
Range("F2").Select
ActiveCell.FormulaR1C1 = "=RC[-2]*RC[-3]"
Selection.AutoFill Destination:=Range("F2:F" & lastrow$)
Range("G2").Select
ActiveCell.FormulaR1C1 = "=SUM(C[-1])"
Selection.Copy
Range("H2").Select
Selection.Insert Shift:=xlDown
Selection.PasteSpecial Paste:=xlValues
Next
```

4–6. Put the products for the actual data in column I, and sum them into J2. Now all we have to do is count the arrangement values that are at least as large. The count is in J3, and the probability in J4.

```
Range("I2").Select
ActiveCell.FormulaR1C1 = "=RC[-6]*RC[-7]"
Selection.AutoFill Destination:=Range("I2:I" & lastrow$)
Range("J2").Select
ActiveCell.FormulaR1C1 = "=SUM(C[-1])"
Range("J3").Select
ActiveCell.FormulaR1C1 = "=COUNTIF(C[-2]:C[-2],"">=""&R[-1]C)"
Range("J4").Select
ActiveCell.FormulaR1C1 = "=(R[-1]C+1)/(2000+1)"
End Sub
```

Glossary

AB design: A phase design with a baseline phase (A) and an intervention phase (B).

ABA design: A phase design with a baseline phase (A), an intervention phase (B), and a withdrawal phase (A).

Absolute value: If we ignore the sign of a number, we are using the absolute value. For example, the absolute value of –3 is 3. The absolute value of +3 is also 3.

Baseline phase: The phase before any intervention or treatment in a phase design.

Blinding: Blinding is concealing which treatment is given from participant or experimenter. Double blinding conceals which treatment is given from both participant and experimenter.

Bootstrap methods: Also known as resampling methods, these assume that the population from which a random sample is drawn has the same form as the random sample, so that an approximation to the population may be obtained by making a very large number of copies of the random sample.

Carry over effect: When a treatment or intervention is withdrawn, there may still be some observable effect of it for some time afterward, and this is known as a carry over effect.

Classification variable: Variables, such as nationality, sex, and political affiliation, that are already a part of a participant and therefore cannot be randomized by the experimenter, are known as classification variables.

Condition: A treatment or combination of treatments assigned to a participant by the experimenter is an experimental condition. In a factorial experiment each combination of factor levels is a condition. For example, in an experiment to investigate two drugs and two relaxation methods, there are four conditions (each drug with each relaxation method).

Confounding: If the effect of a treatment cannot be separated from some other condition, then the effects are said to be confounded. An example would be if all the most seriously ill patients are given the new treatment, whereas those less seriously ill get the regular treatment, then the treatment effect will be confounded with severity of illness. Poor experimental procedures can also cause confounding, for instance if participants on the new treatment get a lot of extra attention.

Conservative (of a test): If the probability of a Type I error is less than the stated size of the test, then the test is said to be conservative because it is less likely than claimed to reject the null hypothesis when it is true.

Effect size: If we compare two treatments or a treatment and control, and the group means are m_a and m_b, the most common measure of effect size is $(m_a - m_b)/sd$ where sd is the common standard deviation. So an effect size will be, for example, half a standard deviation.

External validity: An experiment has external validity if the results can be shown to apply to groups other than the experimental participants. This can be achieved if it is possible to take a random sample from the population of interest, or else by repeating the experiment in different situations and with different types of participant.

Integer: The whole numbers 1, 2, 3, … are the positive integers. There are also negative integers, -1, -2, and so on.

Internal validity: An experiment has internal validity if the effects reported cannot reasonably be attributed to variables or conditions other than the experimental treatments or conditions. If patients on a new experimental treatment are treated by a dedicated team that also provides emotional or social support, whereas control patients attend a standard clinic, internal validity will be compromised because any effect could be due to the additional support given by the dedicated team rather than the experimental treatment.

Intervention phase (in phase designs): All observations from when the intervention is given make up the intervention phase. If the intervention is something like a painkiller, it will be given throughout the intervention phase, but if the intervention is something like a training session or surgery, which is expected to have a permanent or long-lasting effect, then it will be given once and subsequent observations make up the intervention phase.

Macro: A set of instructions that can be reused as many times as needed, usually within a package such as SPSS, Excel, or Word, is known as a macro.

Main effect: In a factorial experiment, the main effect of a factor is the effect of that factor averaged over all levels of other factors. If the factors are type of painkiller (drugs A and B, factor 1) and relaxation method (factor 2), we get the main effect of factor 1 by averaging the drug A response over relaxation methods, and averaging the drug B response over relaxation methods.

Matrix: Numbers arranged in rows and columns form a matrix as long as all rows are the same length and all columns are the same length (data in an Excel or SPSS worksheet often form a matrix).

Monte Carlo methods: These are methods for testing hypotheses (or estimating parameters) that rely on repeated random sampling rather than assumptions about the distribution from which a random sample was taken.

Multiple baseline: Phase designs with more than one participant are called multiple baseline designs. The term may also be used if there is a single participant but more than one measurement at each observation occasion, with an intervention associated with each measurement.

Nonparametric tests: Tests that do not assume a distribution for the measurements from which a random sample is taken are said to be *distribution free* or *nonparametric*.

Nuisance variables: Variables that are not relevant to the experimental design that the experimenter does not and perhaps cannot control but that may affect results are nuisance variables. Examples are the mood or alertness of a participant when they come into the lab to participate in an experiment.

One-tailed test: A test of a null hypothesis against a one-sided alternative that predicts a direction such as "treatment A increases the mean score," as opposed to a two-sided alternative that does not predict a direction such as "treatment A changes the mean score."

Parametric tests: If we assume we know the distribution of measurements from which we take a random sample, for example, that is it a Normal distribution, and we use this assumption about the distribution in our test of a hypothesis about (for instance) the mean of the distribution, then we say we are using a parametric test. ANOVA and the *t* tests are examples.

Partial ordering: The numbers 4, 2, 5, 1, 6, 8 can be arranged in order, but for the numbers 4, 4, 3, 2, 5, 6, 6, where there are ties, only a partial ordering is possible. This may happen in practice at something like a job interview, where two candidates who are better than all the others seem equally good and so occupy joint first place.

Permutation: An arrangement of items is a permutation, for example ABBCA and BACAB are permutations of the letters A, A, B, B, and C.

Phase designs: For each participant, a sequence of observations are taken before any treatment or intervention is given (the baseline phase), then a treatment or intervention is given and observations are continued (the intervention phase). If the intervention does not have a permanent or long-lasting effect there may also be a withdrawal or reversal phase. There may be one or more participants.

Placebo: A treatment (such as a sugar pill) intended to have no effect, given to participants in a control group to conceal from them and the experimenter which treatment they are receiving and to ensure that all participants have the same experience except for the treatment.

Power of a test: The probability of rejecting the null hypothesis when it is in fact false is the power of the test. Phase designs often have rather low power, so even if the intervention does have an effect, the experiment may fail to detect it.

Prebaseline observations: In a phase design, it may be desirable to take measurements on a few occasions before the start of the experimental observations, perhaps to get some insight into the variability to be expected, to allow a stability criterion to be reached, or to decide on the minimum numbers of observations for the phases.

Random nuisance variable: A nuisance variable (such as how tired the participants are) that does not differ systematically among experimental groups is a random nuisance variable. Usually random allocation to experimental groups ensures that any nuisance variables are random nuisance variables.

Random sampling with replacement: Each item selected at random from the population is recorded, then returned to the population before the next item is sampled.

Random sampling without replacement: Each item selected at random from the population is removed from the population so it cannot be drawn again.

Reference set (for a randomization test): The set of test statistics for all possible rearrangements of the data. The reference set would be found by listing all possible rearrangements of the data according to the design and then calculating the test statistic for each of these arrangements. All of these calculated test statistics taken together would then be the reference set. Sometimes we call the arrangements the reference set, as well as the test statistics calculated from them.

Reliability of a measurement: The degree to which a measurement on a participant produces the same result on two occasions, for example, a measurement of height might give high reliability, whereas a measurement of happiness would probably have a lower reliability. Interrater reliability refers to the agreement between two observers who measure the same participant on the same occasion, and is usually an issue when some judgment is required.

Residual sum of squares (RSS): The residual is the difference between an observation and the value predicted for it by an ANOVA, regression, or other model. Squaring and adding the residuals from all the observations give the RSS.

Response guided intervention (in phase designs): If the intervention point is determined by some feature of the baseline observations (such as giving it after four similar observations), we say the intervention is response guided. This differs from determining the intervention point randomly before the start of the experiment, as described for the phase designs in this book.

Reversal: (in phase designs) *see* Withdrawal phase.

Serial correlation: If we have a series of observations on a participant, then observations that are next to each other in the series may be more similar than observations widely separated in the series. This is especially likely if observations are taken at rather short intervals. The tendency of neighboring observations to be similar is called serial correlation.

Simple effect: In a factorial experiment, the effect of factor A at a particular level of factor B is the simple effect of factor A at that level of factor B. Other simple effects are defined in a similar way. For example, in a study where one factor is type of support and the other factor is time of day, one simple effect would be the effect of type of support in the morning, whereas another would be the effect of time of day when there is a high level of support.

Size of a test: The probability of rejecting the null hypothesis when it is in fact true is the size of the test. Typically probabilities of 0.05 or 0.01 are used. So, when we refer to testing at the 0.05 or 5% level, we mean we are using a test of size 0.05.

Sum of products: If we have a pair of measurements (such as height and weight) on each participant, we get the sum of products by multiplying height and weight for each participant and adding the results.

Systematic nuisance variable: Poor experimental design may allow a nuisance variable to be systematic. An example would be if patients are not randomly allocated to a new experimental treatment and a standard one, but instead, the most severely ill patients are allocated to the experimental treatment. Then severity of illness would be a systematic nuisance variable.

Test statistic: A summary of the data designed to exhibit any experimental effect, for instance the difference between two condition means, a count of the number of times something happens or (as in testing order effects) a sum of products. In parametric statistics we use test statistics such as F (ANOVA), t (Student's t), and χ^2. Randomization tests allow freedom to choose an appropriate test statistic for a particular design.

Time series: A sequence of observations on the same participant (or other experimental unit), usually taken at regular intervals, forms a time series. A collection of methods known as time series analysis is available if we have a long series of measurements.

Treatment: In the context of experimental work, a treatment is any condition that the experimenter can give to one or more participants. For example, the term may be used for a drug, a placebo, a training session, or training method.

Truncation: Omitting some of the later digits from a number without rounding is truncation. We often truncate to an integer, so for instance 5.6 may be rounded to the nearest integer (6) but if we truncate it to an integer we get 5.

Two-tailed test: A test of a null hypothesis against a two-sided alternative such as "treatment A changes the mean score" (*see also* One-tailed test).

Type 1 error: If we reject the null hypothesis when it is true, we make a Type 1 error.

Type 2 error: If we fail to reject the null hypothesis when it is false, we make a Type 2 error.

Uniform random number: A random number, which is equally likely to fall anywhere in its range (often 0 to 1), is a uniform random number. So if we have a uniform random number on the interval 0 to 1, it is equally likely to fall above or below 0.5. A random number may also be uniform on a set of integers. For example, if we had a uniform random number on the integers from 5 to 10, it would be equally likely to be 5, 6, 7, 8, 9, or 10.

Washout period: In a repeated measures design, if a treatment or condition has an effect that lasts for some time after being withdrawn, then we need to leave a gap to allow any effect to die away before introducing the next treatment or condition. This gap is the washout period.

Withdrawal phase: If the intervention in a phase design is not permanent or long lasting and there are no ethical reasons why it cannot be withdrawn, then it may be withdrawn to add a withdrawal or reversal phase to the design. *See also* Phase designs.

References

Bulté, I., & Onghena, P. (2008). An R package for single-case randomization tests. *Behavior Research Methods, 4*, 467–478.

Bulté, I., & Onghena, P. (2009). Randomization tests for multiple-baseline designs: An extension of the SCRT-R package. *Behavior Research Methods, 41*, 477–485.

Bulté, I., & Onghena, P. (2011). When the truth hits you between the eyes: A software tool for the visual analysis of single-case experimental data. *Methodology* (in press).

Bulté, I., Van Den Noortgate, W., & Onghena, P. (2010, April). An R package for the nonparametric meta-analysis of small-n educational studies. Poster presented at the annual meeting of the American Educational Research Association (AERA), Denver, CO.

Cohen, J. (1988). *Statistical power analysis for the behavioural sciences* (2nd ed.). Hillsdale, NJ: Lawrence Erlbaum.

Dugard, P., Todman, J., & Staines, H. (2010). Approaching multivariate analysis: a practical introduction (2nd ed.). Hove, UK: Routledge.

Edgington, E. S. (1969). Approximate randomization tests. *The Journal of Psychology, 72*, 143–149.

Edgington, E. S. (1980). *Randomization tests*. New York: Marcel Dekker.

Edgington, E. S., & Onghena, P. (2007). *Randomization tests* (4th ed.). Boca Raton, FL: Chapman Hall/CRC.

Efron, B. (1982). *The jackknife, the bootstrap and other resampling plans*. Bristol: Society for Industrial and Applied Mathematics.

Ferron, J. M., & Sentovich, C. (2002). Statistical power of randomization tests used with multiple baseline designs. *The Journal of Experimental Education, 70*, 165–178.

Ferron, J. M., & Ware, W. B. (1995). Analysing single-case data: the power of randomization tests. *The Journal of Experimental Education, 63*, 167–178.

Fisher, R. A. (1935). *The design of experiments*. Edinburgh: Oliver and Boyd.

Franklin, R. D., Gorman, B. S., Beasley, T. M., & Allison D. B. (1996). Graphical display and visual analysis. In R. D. Franklin, D. B. Allison, & B. S. Gorman (Eds.), *Design and analysis of single case research* (pp. 119–158). Mahwah, NJ: Lawrence Erlbaum.

Howell, D. C. (2010). *Statistical methods for psychology* (7th ed.). Belmont, CA: Wadsworth.

Manly, B. F. J. (2007). *Randomization, bootstrap and Monte Carlo methods in biology* (3rd ed.). Boca Raton, FL: Chapman & Hall/CRC.

Matyas, T. A., & Greenwood, K. M. (1996). Serial dependency in single-case time series. In R. D. Franklin, D. B. Allison, & B. S. Gorman (Eds.), *Design and analysis of single case research* (pp. 215–243). Mahwah, NJ: Lawrence Erlbaum.

McCracken, L. M., Gauntlett-Gilbert, J., & Vowles, K. E. (2007). The role of mindfulness in a contextual cognitive-behavioral analysis of chronic pain-related suffering and disability. *Pain, 131,* 63–69.

Minium, E. W., King, B. M., & Bear, G. (1993). *Statistical reasoning in psychology and education* (3rd ed.). New York: John Wiley.

Morgan, D. L., & Morgan, R. K. (2003). Single-participant research design: Bringing science to managed care. In A. E. Kazdin (Ed.), *Methodological issues and strategies in clinical research* (3rd ed.). Washington DC: American Psychological Association.

Onghena, P. (1994). The power of randomization tests for single-case designs. PhD diss., Katholieke Universiteit Leuven, Belgium.

Onghena, P., & Van Damme, G. (1994). SCRT1.1: Single case randomization tests. *Behaviour Research Methods, Instruments and Computers, 26,* 369.

Primavera, L. H., Allison D. B., & Alfonso V. C. (1997). Measurement of dependent variables. In R. D. Franklin, D. B. Allison, & B. S. Gorman (Eds.), *Design and analysis of single case research* (pp. 41–91). Mahwah, NJ: Lawrence Erlbaum.

Robey, R. R. (2004). A five-phase model for clinical-outcome research. *Journal of Communication Disorders, 37,* 401–411.

Schlosser, R. W. (2009). The Role of Single-Subject Experimental Designs in Evidence-Based Practice Times (National Center for Dissemination of Disability Research Focus Technical Brief No. 22). Austin, TX: National Center for Dissemination of Disability Research. Retrieved from http://www.ncddr.org/kt/products/focus/focus22/

Todman, J., & Dugard, P. (1999). Accessible randomization tests for single-case and small-n experimental designs in AAC research. *Augmentative and Alternative Communication, 15,* 69–82.

Author index

Subject index

Made in the USA
Coppell, TX
26 January 2021